Handbook on
Field Veterinary Surgery

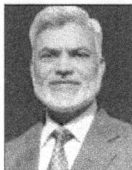

Dr. M.M.S. Zama obtained his professional degree of B.V.Sc & A.H. in 1983 & M.V.Sc. (Vet. Surgery) in 1985 from G. B. Pant University of Agriculture and Technology, Pantnagar. He joined as Assistant Professor (Surgery and Radiology) in December, 1986 at S. K. University of Agricultural Sciences and Technology, Srinagar. During this period, he obtained his Ph.D. degree in 1995 from IVRI, Izatnagar. He was elevated to Associate Professor in 1998 and to Professor in 2006. He joined as Head, Division of Surgery, Indian Veterinary Research Institute, Izatnagar in May, 2009 and as Dean, Faculty of Veterinary Sciences & Animal Husbandry, Sher-e-Kashmir University of Agricultural Sciences & Technology of Jammu in December 2014.

Dr. M. M. S. Zama has a teaching, research, extension and administrative experience of more than 28 years in the University and National Institute. He received National Merit Scholarship, ICAR Junior Research Fellowship, ICAR Senior Fellowship during his studies. He was awarded Vice Chancellor's Gold Medal and Jawaharlal Nehru Trust award for his academic excellence. He co-authored nine laboratory manuals, one guide and one information bulletin for undergraduate students He guided 1 Ph.D. and 5 M.V.Sc. students. He served as member of various interview committees constituted for selection of State Veterinary Officers, Faculty and other staff positions of universities and institute.

Dr. Zama published more than 100 research papers, review and technical articles in international and national journals, received many best paper presentation awards of professional Societies and evaluated research project proposals submitted to DST, DBT, ICMR and CAU, SAUs. During his illustrious career at SKUAST-Jammu and at IVRI, Izatnagar, he has been associated with 13 institute and 3 outside funded research projects in the areas of anaesthesia, physiotherapy, soft tissue surgery, orthopaedic surgery, acellular graft, stem cell therapy and wildlife and made significant contribution in these areas. He along with other scientists patented 4 surgical designs .

Dr. Zama conducted a number of training courses and symposia for the Faculty and Field Veterinarian. He is member of various Sectional Committees of MHDC, Bureau of Indian Standards, New Delhi. He served as Chairman, Board of Studies and the Member of Academic Council, Research Council and Extension Council of the University/Institute. He has delivered many expert lectures and has been referee to various international and national scientific journals. Dr. Zama was elected as Fellow of National Academy of Veterinary Sciences (NAVS) and Indian Society for Veterinary Surgery and is life-member of various Professional Societie**s.**

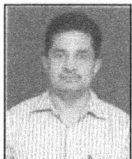

Dr. Hari Prasad Aithal graduated from Veterinary College, Bangalore (1989), and obtained M.V.Sc. (1991) and Ph.D. (1997) degrees from Indian Veterinary Research Institute, Izatnagar (UP). Dr Aithal started his professional career as *Scientist* in the Division of Surgery at IVRI in 1993. Subsequently he was promoted to the post of *Senior Scientist* in 2002, and *Principal Scientist* in the year 2009. During 21 years' of illustrious career, he has been actively involved in research, post-graduate teaching and extension activities. He has been the Principal Investigator or Co-investigator in 20 research projects funded by different agencies. His contribution has been significant in the field of Orthopaedic Surgery and Regional Anaesthesia in ruminants. He has published more than 220 research papers in scientific journals of repute, including 50 papers in renowned International Journals. He has also submitted 02 *Patents* and 06 *Designs* on novel fracture fixation techniques/devices in animals.

Dr. Aithal is the *Associate Editor* of Indian Journal of Veterinary Surgery since 2002, and is an external reviewer for several international and national journals. He has co-edited a Text Book on Anaesthesia and Analgesia for Veterinary Graduates, several Laboratory Manuals, Monograph, Annual Reports, Souvenirs and Compendium of Abstracts. He has been a guide to 4 Ph.D. and 6 M.V.Sc. students, and acted as external examiner for UG/PG courses/thesis evaluation/viva-voce examination of PG students of several universities.

Dr. Aithal has won many awards and honours, including *Best Teacher Award* of the Deemed University, IVRI, Fellowships of the *National Academy of Veterinary Sciences* and *Indian Society for Veterinary Surgery, S.J. Anjelo Memorial Gold Medal* for best paper published in Indian Veterinary Journal, *Dr. A.K. Bhargava Memorial Gold Medal* for the best papers published in Indian Journal of Veterinary Surgery (twice), besides several Best Paper Presentation awards at National Conferences.

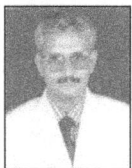

Dr. A.M. Pawde obtained his B.V.Sc. & A.H. in 1987 and M.V.Sc. Vet. Surgery from Nagpur Veterinary College, in 1990. He joined as a scientist at Division of Surgery, IVRI, Izatnagar in 1991. He obtained his PhD degree in 1998. He was recipient of ICAR JRF in 1997 and CSIR SRF in 1994. He was promoted to Senior Scientist in 2000 and Principal Scientist in 2008. He has many awards and honours to his credit including fellowship and best paper presentation of Indian Society for Veterinary Surgery, and Rummy Ramchandran Memorial Gold Medal Award for the best paper published in Indian Veterinary Journal in the field of Oncology (twice) i.e. 1997 and 1999.

Dr. Pawde has been expert member in the committee of wild life, Ministry of Environment & Forests, Indian Bureau of Standards, New Delhi and member, UPPSC, Allahabad, Coordinator, Referral Veterinary Polyclinics, IVRI, Izatnagar. He has been a team member of T'sunami rehabilitation team sent by Director, IVRI. He has delivered many expert lectures, radio talks and TV Interviews. He had been referee to various scientific journals. Dr. Pawde is a life member of various professional societies. During his academic and professional career he actively participated in games, dog shows and horse shows (endurance). He has presented 120 papers and published 110 papers in International and National Journals of repute. Dr. Pawde has the credit of guiding 8 masters and 2 Ph.D. students. During his illustrious career at IVRI he has been associated with nine research project including the Principal Investigator of two projects. He made significant contribution in the areas of veterinary acupuncture with special reference to paralysis in dogs and arthritis in buffaloes.

Handbook on
Field Veterinary Surgery

— Editors —
Dr. M.M.S. Zama
Dr. H.P. Aithal
Dr. A.M. Pawde

2015
Daya Publishing House®
A Division of
Astral International Pvt. Ltd.
New Delhi – 110 002

Cataloging in Publication Data—DK
  Courtesy: D.K. Agencies (P) Ltd. <docinfo@dkagencies.com>

Handbook on field veterinary surgery / editors, Dr. M.M.S.
Zama, Dr. H.P. Aithal, Dr. A.M. Pawde.
    pages ; cm
    Contributed articles.
    Includes index.
    ISBN 978-93-5130-682-5 (International Edition)

    1. Veterinary surgery—India—Handbooks, manuals, etc.   I.
Zama, M. M. S., editor.   II. Aithal, H. P. (Hari Prasad), editor.
III. Pawde, A. M., editor.

DDC 636.08970954   23

| Published by | : | **Daya Publishing House®**
A Division of
Astral International Pvt. Ltd.
– ISO 9001:2008 Certified Company –
4760-61/23, Ansari Road, Darya Ganj
New Delhi-110 002
Ph. 011-43549197, 23278134
E-mail: info@astralint.com
Website: www.astralint.com |
| *Laser Typesetting* | : | **Classic Computer Services**, Delhi - 110 035 |
| *Printed at* | : | **Thomson Press India Limited** |

PRINTED IN INDIA

Dr. Amresh Kumar
B.V.Sc. & A.H., M.V.Sc., Ph.D. (Ill., U.S.A.)
FNAAS, FISVS, FNAVSC
(Ex-Dean, C.VA. Sc., Pantnagar)
Director General, KCMT

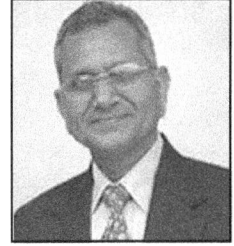

Foreword

I am happy to note that a '*Handbook on Field Veterinary Surgery*' has been edited by Dr. M.M.S. Zama, Dr. H.P. Aithal and Dr. A.M. Pawde. Veterinary Surgery has made significant advancements during last few decades. Surgical operations which were considered difficult to be done in the field, are being commonly performed on animals, be it for disease of eye, heart, lungs, bone and joints, teat and udder; with great ease and success. Non-invasive diagnostic and imaging techniques have revolutionized the diagnosis and treatment of surgical diseases. The fruits of these developments need to be transferred to end users, the live-stock farmers, to increase livestock productivity. This handbook is an attempt ill this direction. The editors have tried to compile the relevant and very useful information on practical aspects of general and operative surgery on recent developments on asepsis and sterilization, suture and suture techniques and basic consideration for surgery. These are to be taken into account to undertake surgery under field consideration, where facilities for major operations are inadequate. Besides practical information on management of surgical diseases, various types of surgical techniques for castration, aural haematoma, ovariohysterectomy, esophagostomy, tracheostomy, hemiorrhaphy, treatment of various types of fractures, foreign body syndrome; and basic eye affections have been written by eminent veterinary surgeons from leading Institutions.

I am confident that this Handbook will prove to be a useful aid for the field veterinary surgeons and will also become a ready reckoner for them. It will surely help in managing the various surgical disorders effectively and efficiently and will reduce livestock morbidity and mortality due to surgical ailments.

I would like to congratulate Dr. M.M.S. Zama, Dr. H.P. Aithal and Dr. A.M. Pawde (Editors) for publication of this Handbook on Field Veterinary Surgery. I wish them good luck for all their endeavours.

Amresh Kumar
Director General
KCMT

Preface

The number of surgical conditions being reported in veterinary hospitals is ever increasing due to changing socioeconomic status of urban as well as rural India, growing industrialization, increased vehicular traffic and also greater awareness among the livestock and pet owners about the treatment options available. Though the modern advanced techniques, facilities and expertise are available in established veterinary institutes and college hospitals across the country, most of the time they are beyond the reach of a common man. Many a times, animal owners expect their animals to be treated at their doorstep, wherein the role of field veterinary surgeon becomes important. Relatively less expertise and technical assistance available, coupled with poor veterinary infrastructure and facilities at village levels make the job of a field veterinarian challenging and demanding. Apart from attending general health problems of livestock, he is also expected to treat common surgical conditions routinely encountered in animal patients.

With the advent of newer diagnostic and surgical techniques, which can be adapted in field conditions, along with easy access to internet facility at every remote corner, the face of field surgery is changing. Further, more and more postgraduates, especially from clinical disciplines are entering into field service, making it possible to undertake specialized surgeries at the field level. Many surgical conditions can be treated in the field by maintaining minimum standards of surgery with least facility; mostly it is the confidence and skill of the surgeon that determine the outcome of a surgical intervention. In order to develop confidence and surgical skill, however, one has to keep abreast with the latest developments in the related areas of diagnostic imaging like X-rays and ultrasonography, anaesthetic protocols, and surgical techniques. Though there are several text books which describe different surgical techniques, they are very exhaustive and not readily accessible to a field vet. Hence, there was a need to have a hand book, which can act as ready reference for the field veterinary surgeons, describing simple surgical techniques which are easy to understand and practice.

The contents of this book are specially designed keeping in view the needs of veterinary surgeons working at the field level. The book provides concise but comprehensive hands on information on a variety of surgical conditions commonly encountered in different domestic animals. The contents have been written from different authors, who are experienced surgeons and teachers engaged in day to day clinical practice, and are experts in the particular field. The book contains the basic information, and the techniques are described in simple language, which can be easily understood by a veterinary surgeon with limited subject knowledge.

The handbook contains 23 chapters comprising almost all the surgical conditions encountered in the field. Prospects and basic considerations in field level surgery, methods of sterilization, suturing techniques and materials are comprehensively described in the initial chapters. Common surgical techniques like management of wounds, tumours, urolithiasis, castration in different species of animals, ovariohysterectomy in bitches and caesarean section in large animals have been described in subsequent chapters. This was followed by specific soft tissue surgeries like oesophagotomy, tracheotomy/tracheostomy, foreign body syndrome, intestinal surgery, hernia repair, rectal prolapse, atresia ani and recti, which have been detailed considering their importance in the field level. Simple techniques for management of horn injuries, bone fractures, tendon injuries, patellar desmotomy and foot affections are described in the following chapters. At the end, surgery of teat, ear haematoma and eye affections have been covered. The chapters on different surgical conditions describe basic considerations, instrumentation, anaesthesia, surgical technique, and pre- and post-operative care of animals with the help of diagrams or/and photographs. More emphasis was given to the easy-to-do surgical techniques, which are common and can be performed at the field level with limited facilities and assistance. Hence the book is a ready reference to all the field veterinary surgeons and fresh veterinary graduates who wish to pursue their career as veterinary surgeons in the field. The hand book can play a great role in updating the knowledge, building confidence and refreshing the skill of the field veterinarians. We hope that the book will help in bringing a perceptible change in the field veterinary surgery in days to come.

We earnestly thank all the contributors who have contributed chapters in the book, without their active support it would not be possible to bring out this compilation.

Dr. M.M.S. Zama
Dr. H.P. Aithal
Dr. A.M. Pawde

Contents

List of Contributors

Aithal, H.P.
Principal Scientist, Division of Surgery, Indian Veterinary Research Institute, Izatnagar, U.P.

Amarpal
Principal Scientist, Division of Surgery, Indian Veterinary Research Institute, Izatnagar, U.P.

Athar, Hakim
Associate Professor (Surgery), Faculty of Veterinary Sciences & AH., SKUAST-Jammu, J&K

Bhardwaj, H.R.
Associate Professor (Surgery), Faculty of Veterinary Sciences & AH., SKUAST-Jammu, J&K

Chaudhary, R.N.
Assistant Professor (Surgery), COVS, LLRUVAS, Hisar, Haryana

Devi, Kh. Sangeeta
Associate Professor, College of Veterinary Sciences & AH, NDU&AT, Kumarganj, Faizabad, U.P.

Fazili, M.R.
Associate Professor (Surgery), Faculty of Veterinary Sciences & AH., SKUAST-Jammu, J&K

Gangwar, A.K.
Associate Professor, College of Veterinary Sciences & AH, NDU&AT, Kumarganj, Faizabad, U.P.

Gopinathan, Aswathy
Scientist, Division of Surgery, Indian Veterinary Research Institute, Izatnagar, U.P.

Gupta, Ajay Kumar
Associate Professor (Surgery), Faculty of Veterinary Sciences & AH., SKUAST-Jammu, J&K

Hoque, Mozammel
Principal Scientist, Division of Surgery, Indian Veterinary Research Institute, Izatnagar, U.P.

Kinjavdekar, Prakash
Principal Scientist, Division of Surgery, Indian Veterinary Research Institute, Izatnagar, U.P.

Maiti, S.K.
Principal Scientist, Division of Surgery, Indian Veterinary Research Institute, Izatnagar, U.P.

Mohindroo, J.
Associate Professor (Surgery), College of Veterinary Sciences, GADVASU, Ludhiana, Punjab

Moulvi, B.A.
Professor and Head (Surgery), Faculty of Veterinary Sciences & AH., SKUAST-Jammu, J&K

Pathak, Rekha
Senior Scientist, Division of Surgery, Indian Veterinary Research Institute, Izatnagar, U.P.

Pawde, A.M.
Principal Scientist, Division of Surgery, Indian Veterinary Research Institute, Izatnagar, U.P.

Saxena, Abhishek Chandra
Scientist, Division of Surgery, Indian Veterinary Research Institute, Izatnagar, U.P.

Sharma, A.K.
Principal Scientist, Division of Surgery, Indian Veterinary Research Institute, Izatnagar, U.P.

Singh, Gaj Raj
Former Head, Division of Surgery, Indian Veterinary Research Institute, Izatnagar and Former Dean, College of Veterinary Sciences & A.H. Selesih, Aizawl, Mizoram

Singh, Harnam
Dean, College of Veterinary Sciences & AH, NDU&AT, Kumarganj, Faizabad, U.P.

Singh, Kiranjeet
Senior Scientist, Division of Surgery, Indian Veterinary Research Institute, Izatnagar, U.P.

Sivanarayanan, T.B.
Ph.D. Scholar, Division of Surgery, Indian Veterinary Research Institute, Izatnagar, U.P.

Tyagi, S.P.
Associate Professor, Department of Surgery and Radiology, CSKHPAU, Palampur, H.P.

Zama, M.M.S.
Professor and Head, Division of Surgery, Indian Veterinary Research Institute, Izatnagar, U.P.

1

Prospects and Recent Advances in Field Level Surgery in Livestock

M.M.S. Zama

From the start of civilization, human beings have utilized different animal species for a variety of purposes *viz.* food, apparel, drought power, companionship, entertainment, research experimentation, security etc. Livestock wealth is deemed as the oldest wealth resource for mankind and is still considered as a symbol of economic status in the rural society. Livestock sector plays a significant role in the Indian economy. Contribution of livestock to agricultural gross domestic product (Ag GDP) has been rising; it increased from 14 per cent in 1980-81 to 24.7 per cent in 2009-10 (MoA, 2011). Of the total household in the rural area, about 73 per cent own some form of livestock.

Increasing colonization, industrialization and traffic has lead to a drastic increase in the surgical affections of the livestock. As most of the livestock owners are small and marginal farmers, such problems add to the economic burden on already overloaded farmers. Veterinary surgeons are not directly concerned with the production aspect of livestock but surgical interventions are many a times required to salvage or prolong the life of an animal having good production potential or to improve the work efficiency of drought animals. Sometimes palliative surgery is required to reduce the sufferings of the animal. Because of the obvious constraints associated with transport, handling and restraint of livestock species together with the poor veterinary infrastructure in rural India, which is the principal beneficiary, role of veterinary surgeons becomes very challenging and demanding. Most of the times, animal owners want veterinary aid at their doorstep.

Field veterinarians successfully deal with many minor surgical affections in livestock, like opening an abscess or cyst, castration, shearing of over grown horn, application of plaster cast and suturing of wound. However, surgical interventions like amputation of tail, suturing teat fistula, caesarean section, fracture management, amputation of horn, urethrotomy, cystotomy, removal of eye worm, rumenotomy, amputation of rectal or vaginal prolapse, patellar desmotomy, modified gastrocnemius tenectomy and excision of tumour etc. require a great level of confidence and skill.

Various problems associated in the diagnosis and management of surgical affections at field level include:

☆ Lack of proper infrastructure such as operation theatre, protective clothing, aseptic techniques, availability and accessibility of basic surgical instruments and sterilization facilities.

☆ Lack of proper diagnostic modalities such as radiography, ultrasonography and fluoroscopy etc.

☆ Most of the surgical interventions in livestock involve higher cost which overrides the economic value of the animal.

☆ Post-operative management and care of the animal is difficult due to lack of knowledge and ignorance on the part of farmer.

☆ Availability of life saving and emergency drugs is limited as they are rarely used and are costly.

☆ Lack of skilled staff necessary for assistance during various surgical interventions.

☆ Most of the animals are presented in advanced conditions (*e.g.* caesarean section) due to the lack of knowledge regarding seriousness of the problem.

However, with recent developments in the field of veterinary clinical sciences, a new era is in its phase of inception, where high quality diagnostic and therapeutic modalities will be available to the animal owners at the remotest of villages at substantially affordable prices. Portable hand held X-ray machines can be taken to the farmer's doorstep for proper diagnosis of fracture cases. With the help of internet, the radiographs can be shared with a specialist sitting far away in any corner of the country for diagnosis and advice on surgical intervention.

Ultrasound once considered as a luxury has now emerged as the most versatile diagnostic imaging modality. Portable, battery operated ultrasound machines with advanced imaging options like colour and pulse Doppler are available at highly affordable prices and are being installed at State Veterinary Facilities. They can not only revolutionize the diagnostic services at field level, but can also significantly improve the accuracy of pregnancy diagnosis in livestock, which can be a boon to the farmers. Cases of reduced reproductive performance can be diagnosed very efficiently with ultrasound examination and this will not only help in proper management of such cases but also drastically reduce the cost of treatment.

Laparoscopy and endoscopic machines have also become affordable and if installed at District level, they can work wonders in cases where it is difficult to access and image an organ. Animals suffering from conditions like oesophageal or tracheal obstruction, intestinal obstruction etc. can be very efficiently managed with these techniques. Imaging techniques like CT scan and MRI are still farfetched things in the veterinary field but one day they will be as easily accessible to veterinary patients as they are to human patients today.

Surgical techniques have also come a long way in recent years. Many advances have taken place in the areas of gastrointestinal, respiratory, urogenital, cardiovascular, ophthalmic, orthopaedic and neurosurgery. Animals suffering from urinary obstruction were doomed as surgery was considered very difficult in field conditions, but newer techniques like tube cystostomy has emerged as a life saver for these animals without taxing the veterinarian, animal or its owner. Compound fractures almost always rendered the animal unproductive but with the advent of newer techniques of external skeletal fixation which can be customized according to the size of animal and site of fracture, this condition can be successfully managed most of the time. Another advantage of these techniques is their cost effectiveness and they do not put much economic burden on the livestock owners.

Hernia is a very commonly encountered condition in large animals at field conditions. Most of them can be corrected with the help of conventional treatment techniques, but sometimes they are either too big to be repaired conventionally or the surrounding muscles are too weak to hold the sutures. In such cases use of grafts is warranted. Research on this line is already on and the day is not far when xenogenic, non-immunogenic, ready to use grafts for veterinary patients will be commercially available at affordable price. Advanced treatment techniques, like total hip joint replacement, lens transplantation etc., are also done more frequently in India.

Newer treatment concepts like use of healing promoters, mesenchymal stem cells and cell seeded implants are also finding their way in the routine treatment of various surgical disorders like fractures, dislocations, burn injuries, osteoarthritis and nerve injuries. These techniques are easy to use, and with slight modifications can be used at field level. In the near future they may also appear in ready to use packages for direct application.

Physiotherapy is one of the fastest developing fields in the veterinary as well as medical sciences. Research on newer physiotherapeutic modalities like interferential nerve muscle stimulation, static magnetic therapy, diathermy, electro-acupuncture etc. have shown some promising results in various conditions affecting different animal species. Physiotherapy is not solely indicated in neuromuscular disorders but it can be used for rehabilitation of surgical patients, thereby reducing their sufferings and time of functional recovery. These modalities are not very costly and can be easily applied at the field level with minimal training and expertise.

Surgery is an ever evolving field and newer advances are frequently overcoming the limitations of field level surgery but basic principles of surgery as stated by Halsted still stand true. Surgery at field level is probably more dependent on the will power and self confidence of the surgeon. Veterinary facilities at the field are fast improving and it is the duty of the veterinarians to keep pace with these changes through continual improvement in their professional competence and skill and keeping abreast of recent advances.

2

Basic Considerations for Field Level Surgery

Gaj Raj Singh

The veterinarians are expected to help the community to make use of animal resources fully and in a sustainable manner. Therefore, a veterinarian is supposed to perform several tasks such as handling, examining and treating all species of animals; carrying diagnostic tests including X-rays and ultrasound scans; immunizing animals against different types of diseases; performing surgery including managing anaesthesia; maintaining up to date records and many other nondescript tasks. In order to perform these tasks effectively, he/she has to keep himself/herself abreast with the latest technical developments in different areas including surgical techniques, X-rays, ultrasound and anaesthetic protocols. Therefore, continuing education can play great role in updating the knowledge and refreshing the skill of the field veterinarians.

The basic principles of surgery are the same for pet and farm animals. The goal of veterinary surgery are, however, quite different in pets and in farm animals. In the former situation, surgery is a bit like in human beings, and more and more complex operations are performed, with sophisticated anaesthesia techniques. The Small Animal Surgery involves providing the highest quality care available. Facilities such as ultrasonography, digital radiography, computed tomography, and magnetic resonance imaging to aid in diagnosis of pet's condition are now used in veterinary practice. Advanced surgical treatments, including repair of complicated fractures, minimally invasive surgery (arthroscopy and laparoscopy) and spinal surgery are now available for pets.

In farm animals, which we deal at field level, the techniques used for small animals can be practiced; however, the cost of the operation must not exceed the economic benefit in surgically treating the illness. Therefore, while planning the basic requirements for field level surgery, one has to maintain standards of surgery yet keep the cost of surgery within limits for positive outcome.

The clinics designed to function in the remote areas require attention to minimally acceptable standards to adequately and safely perform surgery. Although specific protocols may vary depending upon many factors, there exists a minimally acceptable level which all clinics should mandate. This ensures safety and well-being of animals and clinical staff, and maintains quality controls over service delivered. The standard applied to the patient on the day of surgery will affect the immediate outcome of the patient as well as long after the patient has recovered from surgery. Minimally acceptable standards should be established, met and followed for each specific programme. It is important that all the staff acknowledge the seriousness of anaesthesia and surgery on every individual patient.

General Considerations

☆ Surgery is a team work; therefore, communication with the local veterinary community in the area may enhance the overall effectiveness and outcome of the surgery.

☆ The language skills are imperative for communication. If you can speak in local language that may help in understanding the case and in giving proper post-operative direction to the owner.

☆ You should know your case. Surgery should not be considered as luxury, way to demonstrate your ability, earn money or impress others. One should decide to undertake the surgery when it is the only option left to treat the case. Otherwise, it may prove disastrous if wrong decision is taken. In cases where surgery is unavoidable, it should be planned and executed as early as possible.

☆ You should know yourself. Have you operated such cases earlier? Are you prepared to meet any complication that may arise during surgery? If yes, go ahead with confidence. If not, do not hesitate referring the case to the nearest clinic, where facilities for operating such cases are available or request a friend, who is competent to operate the case. Read the surgical procedure carefully in a good book prior to operating the case.

☆ You should know your facilities. Make the list of inventories needed during surgery and emergency. If anything is missing, it is better to arrange well in advance before the start of surgery.

☆ Check the cleanliness. Although surgery can be performed anywhere, cleanliness of the area should be established and maintained as best as possible. Operations often performed outdoors yet should not excuse attention to cleanliness. Address cleanliness prior to the start of any surgery.

☆ Check whether running water supply is available or not. If not arrange/ obtain adequate water holding container for cleaning of instruments, preparation of patient and surgery team, cleaning of table etc.

☆ Check for the availability of electricity. If no electricity is available or there is possibility of power breakdown, arrange suitable power backup for equipments.

☆ Check for lighting. If the natural light on the site is sufficient. Adjunct lighting should be available for early morning, late afternoon or evening surgery and cloudy days.

☆ Protection from sun, rain and wind must be addressed if surgery is performed outdoors.

☆ During winter additional source of heat may be needed to be supplied for surgery, recovery or ill cases.

☆ Facilities for trash collection and disposal and for disposal of biohazard material.

☆ Spays and castrations are almost elective procedures. The risks versus the benefit of surgery must be considered in each case with the final decision with the owner.

Pre-Surgery Meeting

It is always advisable to arrange an additional meeting with all the team to discuss analgesic, anaesthetic and surgical protocols, emergency protocols and approach to possible surgical complications.

Sterilization of Surgical Instruments and Supplies

Sterilization of surgical instruments and supplies is an essential component for successful outcome of the surgery. Method to sterilize instruments and supplies should be determined in advance of the surgery. Many veterinary hospitals/ dispensaries may not have access to autoclave although they may have access to pressure cooker. An autoclave or pressure cooker will kill all the viable organisms including spores when done at the correct time and temperature (121degree centigrade at 15 pound pressure for 30 minutes). Autoclaves are expensive and usually difficult to maintain or repair in remote locations. Pressure cookers lend themselves well to remote work. They are relatively cheap and easy to maintain. They can be purchased either electric or gas.

Although steam sterilization is recognized as the preferred method of sterilization of equipment and supplies, chemical disinfection, when proper instructions are followed, is an acceptable method for disinfecting instruments for surgical procedures. Disinfecting solutions kill most microorganisms except spores when done properly and according to manufacturer's recommendations. It is important to understand the chemical properties of the specific disinfecting solution in order to avoid side effects such as chemical peritonitis. There is a large product list based on germicidal activity (high to low). Several commercial products such as Cidex, Benz All or Surgical Crit are available. Minimally acceptable standards for chemical disinfection are:

☆ Solution prepared to manufacturer's instructions

☆ Instruments clean and dried

☆ Total immersion

☆ Unclamped

☆ Timed according to manufacturer's instructions

☆ Removed with sterile haemostat

Records

A record is required on every animal admitted to the clinic. Records provide a written log of patient, owner data and physical parameters with which to decide if the animal is a surgical candidate. Feral or extremely aggressive animals must have a record even if they cannot be examined prior to sedation and/or anaesthesia and their status noted on the record. Feral or extremely aggressive animals are examined after sedation or anaesthesia, prior to surgery.

Physical Examination

All animals must receive a physical examination prior to undergoing anaesthesia and surgery. Exceptions to this will be feral or extremely aggressive animals. Often field clinics are held in impoverished areas. A record and physical examination demonstrates the care, dedication and respect each animal receives and establishes a good reputation within the community. This in turn often increases the value and worth of the animal in the owner's eyes and the value of the veterinarian in the community's eyes.

Many animals in field may not be in the best of health. Often no preoperative diagnostics are available. A good physical examination may identify potential problems which can be addressed accordingly, minimizing complications. The findings on physical examination will determine the appropriate anaesthetic and surgical protocols. Pediatric, geriatric, pregnant or metabolically compromised animal will need special planning.

Minimal Data to be Recorded

☆ Temperature.

☆ Pulse rate and quality.

☆ Respiration rate and lung sounds.

☆ Capillary refill time and mucous membrane colour and texture.

☆ Examination of all other systems for clinically relevant findings.

☆ An accurate weight is needed to calculate the correct dose of any medication to be administered. A baby scale or fish scale can be used in animals under 4.5 kilograms. Aweight scale can be used for animals greater than 4.5 kilograms.

☆ It is also important to consider body condition score (BCS) with regard to analgesic and anaesthetic dosing. Certain medications, especially anaesthetics, are more accurately dosed and are metabolized based on lean body weight versus overall body weight. Experienced staff should assign a BCS score to more effectively address analgesia and anaesthesia.

Food and Water

Normal preoperative instructions are to withhold food for eight hours prior to admission to the clinic. It is not needed, nor recommended to withhold water prior to admission, especially as the environment of a field clinic can contribute to dehydration.

Paediatrics

Paediatric patients are defined as a patient less than 16 weeks of age. Although normal pre-operative instructions are to withhold food for 8 hours prior to surgery, paediatric patients are the exception to this advice. They are much more prone to hypoglycaemia. They may not be taken to surgery for hours after presentation. Their complete eating history may not be known. Paediatric patients should be fed two to four hours prior to surgery. If surgery is done within two hours of presentation, their blood glucose level can be augmented by giving honey. Glucose/dextrose solutions should never be given by any other route than intravenously or orally.

Thermoregulation

Ambient temperatures in a field clinic can range from extremely cold to very hot. Anaesthesia and surgery disrupt the normal thermoregulatory mechanisms and typically cause the patient to become cold. Inattention to thermoregulation of the patient produces significant and often avoidable complications and it is the most common post-operative complication. Methods to address thermoregulation include:

☆ Monitoring temperatures intra-operatively and in recovery.

☆ The use of a digital thermometer in the nostril intra-op gives a general idea of body temperature.

☆ Placing material between the animal and table surface such as newspaper, bubble wrap or a dry towel.

☆ Warm, ambient temperatures are not conveyed to the table surface. The material of the table surface may contribute to an already disrupted thermoregulatory mechanism.

☆ Cool or cold ambient temperatures can worsen this and may require additional attention to thermoregulation. In addition, heat loss from an animal to the table surface can be significant, even if the ambient temperature is high. This is especially important in cats, small dogs and paediatric patients.

☆ Keep patients warm and dry. Wet animals are much more prone to hypothermia.

☆ Keep heat sources available such as socks filled with rice and warmed in a microwave, warm water bottles, heating pads etc.

☆ Never put a heat source directly against an animal's skin as they are very easy to burn.

☆ Minimize the use of water and cold prep solutions. Excess prep liquid should not be squeezed on to the surgical surface. Alcohol greatly and rapidly lowers body temperature. Routine use is not recommended.

☆ Intravenous or subcutaneous fluids. Fluids at room temperature are colder than a normal animal's body temperature and can contribute to hypothermia. Warm subcutaneous fluids may help address hypothermia.

☆ Room temperature subcutaneous fluids may help address hyperthermia.

☆ If working in an extremely hot environment with minimal to no ventilation, employ methods to keep body temperatures within acceptable parameters. Use fans, cool floors, IV fluids, cool water bottles.

Emergency Preparation

☆ Sterilizations in any setting, but especially in a field setting, can be complicated. Every clinic should be prepared to address emergencies or complications that may arise. Emergency drugs and procedures should be established and discussed prior to the start of the clinic. Additional items to have on hand include:

☆ Endotracheal tubes and laryngoscope. A recognized veterinary professional and the equipment and technical skill must be available to insert an endotracheal tube in an emergency situation.

☆ Ambu bag is essential for assisted breathing if no oxygen is available.

☆ Often available free from human hospitals.

☆ Emergency drugs such as atropine, epinephrine and any reversal agents. Diphenhydramine and dexamethasone should be on hand in case of acute anaphylactic reactions.

☆ Intravenous catheters

☆ Intravenous fluids

☆ The ability to address thermoregulation

☆ Additional anaesthetics and pain medications

☆ A chart of emergency drug doses by weight so as to minimize time performing calculations

Surgical Risk Patients

Cases presented in field surgeries are often more of a surgical risk. The desire to address as many animals as possible is certainly a goal but should not come at the expense of individual cases. Patients deemed to be high risk should be discussed with the owner prior to the procedure and also need final approval from the veterinarian of record prior to admission. These include paediatric, pregnant, physically or metabolically compromised, or geriatric patients. Sometimes it is in the best interest of the animal to not perform a surgery.

Minimum Surgeon Knowledge Base

☆ Knowledge of the common anaesthetics and analgesics and their antidotes

☆ Knowledge of surgical procedure to be performed

☆ Identify and understand the use of surgical instruments and materials

☆ Ability to tie secure ligatures (square, surgeon's knots)

☆ Anatomy of the surgical procedure. Allows identification of normal versus abnormal anatomy and how to surgically address differences.

☆ Peri-surgical skills

☆ Recognize contamination and how to respond

☆ Know how to isolate structures to find the source of haemorrhage and apply

☆ Recognize complications and know how to respond

☆ Recognize the haemorrhage, primary due to surgical complications, secondary due to disease and/or parasites.

Conclusions

Lack of adherence to minimal standards can adversely affect the patient's outcome. While undertaking surgery every step including decision to undertake surgery, preparation for surgery, induction and maintenance of anaesthesia, surgical procedure, and recovery and post-operative rehabilitation is important. It is often a difficult, time consuming and sometimes frustrating process. Proper planning can certainly help address all of the above.

3

Asepsis and Sterilization

Hakim Athar and B.A. Moulvi

Principles of Surgical Asepsis

Sterilization is the complete destruction of micro-organisms (bacteria, viruses and spores) on items like surgical instruments, implants, drapes, catheters, needles and attire that come in contact with tissue or enter the vascular system.

Disinfection is the destruction of most pathogenic micro-organisms on inanimate (non-living) objects, whereas *antisepsis* is the destruction of most pathogenic micro-organisms on animate (living) objects.

Antiseptics are used to kill micro-organisms during patient skin preparation and surgical scrubbing, however, the skin is not sterilized. *Cleaning* is the removal of foreign materials (*e.g.* soil, organic material, micro-organisms) from objects and surfaces and is normally accomplished by the use of water, mechanical action and detergents. It may be manual or mechanical, using ultrasonic cleaners or washer/disinfectors that may facilitate cleaning and decontamination of some items and reduce the need for handling. Thorough cleaning is essential before high-level disinfection and sterilization because inorganic and organic materials that remain on the surfaces of instruments interfere with the effectiveness of these processes. Although cleaning does remove soil and bacteria, it does not kill or inactivate viruses. Decontamination is a process which removes or destroys micro-organisms to render an object safe for use

Aseptic technique is defined as the method and practice that prevent cross contamination during surgery. It involves proper preparation of the facilities and environment, surgical site, surgical team, surgical equipments and instruments.

Infection first requires micro-organisms being introduced into the surgical wound. The source of the micro-organisms may be exogenous (*i.e.*, the air, surgical instruments, surgical team or patient) or endogenous (*i.e.*, organisms that originate in the patient's body). It is impossible to eliminate all micro-organisms from the surgical wound and sterile the surgical field, however, aseptic technique limits the patient's exposure to a number of micro-organisms that are detrimental.

Prevention of Surgical Infections

Prevention of surgical site infection requires attention to numerous factors. They include:

Preparation of Patient for Surgery

Before surgery, the patient should be examined for evidence of bacterial infection, including evaluation of the skin and urinary tract, and surgery is postponed pending resolution of infection if possible. The patient's skin is cleaned preoperatively to reduce surgical site contamination. As skin can not be sterilized, it is usually the weakest link in the maintenance of sterile surgical field. Preparation of the surgical site should include hair removal and cleansing to remove gross contamination, dirt and oil, and to reduce resident skin flora prior to antiseptic skin preparation. Shaving of hair is avoided because it causes multiple lacerations and skin erosions that are rapidly colonized by bacteria. Clipping is done immediately before the surgery and not a day before.

Surgical scrubs are applied to the area starting at the expected surgical incision and moving outward in expanding concentric circles, moving towards the periphery. This manoeuvre is repeated, alternating rinse solutions with the antiseptic until the sponges are free of visible soiling. Overzealous scrubbing should be avoided as it brings bacteria from within the hair follicles to the surface and causes irritation and abrasions that are rapidly invaded by bacteria. Then a final application of the disinfectant is done and left in place. Commonly used preparations are tinctures of chlorhexidene and iodine.

Surgical drapes should prevent the movement of debris and bacteria from non-sterile areas onto the surgical field for the duration of surgery. They should be economical, easy to sterilize and should retain their barrier properties if they are washed, sterilized and reused. Cotton muslin drapes are routinely used in veterinary practice. However, they lose their effectiveness once they become wet and can allow passage of bacteria through them (strikethrough).

Preparation of the Surgical Team

The operating team consists of the people administering anaesthesia, performing surgery, non-scrubbed assistant and observers within the operating room. All of them contribute to the operating room contamination and potential infection of the wound. Careful preparation of the surgical team and non-sterile personnel reduces the number of bacteria in the surgical suite. A correlation has been noted between the number of people, their movements, and the number of airborne bacteria in a surgical suite. Therefore, scrub suits, caps, masks, sweat bands, shoe covers, gowns and gloves are worn to prevent shed particulates and micro-organisms from reaching the surgery site.

The objective of a surgical hand scrub is to remove gross dirt and oil, and decrease bacterial counts, and to have a prolonged depressant effect on transient and resident microflora of the hands and forearms. It should not be time consuming and should not irritate the skin.

Surgical scrub protocols are based either on scrubbing time or on stroke counting. Fingernails are kept short, clean and free of polish and artificial nails. Jewellery should be removed. All surfaces of the hands and forearms below the elbow are exposed to antiseptic scrub. Special attention is paid to the area under the nails. The ideal scrub time is unknown, but 2 to 5 minutes seems to be safe and effective, depending on the agent used.

Gloves are worn by the operating team to protect the patient from the micro-organisms on the operating team's skin. They also protect the operating team from the patient's micro-organisms.

Preparation of the Operating Facilities

There should be separate induction, preparation and recovery rooms. The operating room should provide an environment as free as possible from bacterial contamination. Floors and walls should be surfaced so that cleaning is efficient, and drains should be placed so that water does not pool anywhere in the surgical suite after cleaning. All the surfaces in the operating room should be carefully disinfected daily, and the tables are disinfected in between operations. Operating room doors should remain closed during the surgery, and traffic through the room should remain minimal. Air within the operating room should be under mild positive pressure, so that when the doors open, air flows out of the room rather than into it.

Common Antiseptic Agents

Alcohols

Alcohols kill bacteria by coagulation of proteins. Ethanol is generally used as a 70 per cent solution and isopropyl alcohol is effective in concentration of up to 99 per cent. Alcohols are effective only against vegetative bacteria, and have poor activity against viruses and spores. When alcohol is allowed to stand in open containers, alcohol decreases in concentration and at lower concentration, they become bacteriostatic rather than bactericidal. Alcohols are inactivated by a variety of organic debris and have no residual activity after evaporation. Alcohols have higher and more rapid kill rate than chlorhexidine, and third best is povidone-iodine.

Chlorhexidine

Chlorhexidine binds to protein of the stratum corneum, forming a persistent residue that can kill bacteria emerging from sebaceous glands, sweat glands and hair follicles during surgery. It is non-irritant to the skin and its effectiveness increases after repeated use. It is available in detergent, tincture and aqueous form. It is effective against gram positive and gram negative organisms. Chlorhexidine (0.02 per cent), like 1 per cent povidone-iodine, promotes intra-abdominal adhesion formation and therefore should not be used for peritoneal lavage.

Iodine Compounds

Inorganic or elemental iodine has a very broad antimicrobial spectrum compared with other agents and a very short kill time at low concentrations, and organisms do not develop resistance to it. Its undesirable characteristics are odour, tissue irritation, staining, radiopacity and corrosiveness. Concentration greater than 3.5 per cent is toxic to tissues and does not provide additional disinfectant activity. Iodophors are complexes of elemental iodine with a carrier, such as polyvinylpyrrolidone (PVP), which forms povidone-iodine. Before application of iodophor compounds, hair should be removed and the skin well cleaned to remove organic debris that can reduce the bactericidal activity of the iodophor.

Phenols

Phenol or carbolic acid is the oldest known germicidal agent. Hexachlorophene has a relatively slow onset of action but a prolonged residual activity, and it is not adversely affected by organic materials. Phenols are bactericidal but do not affect viruses and spores. Hexachlorophene based preparations are inactivated by alcohol. Use was largely curtailed after hexachlorophene was shown to be neurotoxic at levels obtained with dermal exposure.

Quaternary Ammonium Compounds

Quaternary ammonium compounds, such as benzalkonium chloride, are cationic surfactants that dissolve lipids in bacterial cell walls and membranes. They are effective against both gram positive and gram negative bacteria. Disadvantages are ineffectiveness against viruses, spores and fungi, formation of residue layers, and inactivation by common organic debris and soaps.

Sterilization of Surgical Equipment/Instruments

Any equipment or supplies that come in contact with body tissues or blood must be sterile. The methods of the sterilization can be broadly divided into two groups, physical and chemical. Dry heat, moist heat (boiling and steam treatment), filtration, ionizing radiation (gamma and electron beam radiation) and plasmas are commonly used physical methods. Chemical sterilization is accomplished with ethylene oxide, hydrogen peroxide, formaldehyde, ozone gases or β-propiolactone.

Commonly used sterilization processes have a variety of advantages and disadvantages. For example, the steam autoclave, a 200-year-old sterilization technology, is an effective sterilization process, but its high temperature and moisture make it unusable for many of today's devices. Likewise, dry-heat sterilization has process temperatures that cannot be tolerated by most devices.

Low-temperature, low-moisture processes, such as sterilization by ETO gas or hydrogen peroxide gas plasma, are used for many medical devices. Increasingly, operating room (OR) personnel are being asked to sterilize equipment more quickly and efficiently and with lower cost. Advanced sterilization systems that enable more rapid availability of wrapped, sterile devices and instruments may result in more rapid turnover of the OR suite and less "downtime" between procedures. Swift and efficient sterilization of expensive heat-and moisture-sensitive medical and surgical devices (*i.e.*, cameras, fiberoptic cables and rigid endoscopes) is particularly advantageous when costs of such equipment may limit their duplication in most veterinary practices. A low-temperature hydrogen peroxide gas plasma sterilization system that provides terminal sterilization of sophisticated instruments in 55 minutes is useful for such devices.

Physical Methods

Thermal Energy

Steam sterilization is nontoxic, inexpensive, rapidly microbicidal, sporicidal, and rapidly heats and penetrates fabrics. The temperature range within which micro-organisms survive is largely determined by the thermal viability of their proteins and nucleic acids. Dry heat kills micro-organisms by reacting with and oxidizing their proteins, while in moist heat the microbial proteins undergo denaturation, a process in which the three-dimensional form of the protein reverts to a two-dimensional form, and the protein breaks down. Moist heat in the form of pressurized steam is regarded as the practical and dependable method for the destruction of all forms of life, including bacterial spores. The denaturation or destruction of the cellular protein is the principal means by which heat destroys micro-organisms. A critical relationship between temperature, pressure and exposure time required to kill the microbes is the function of their individual heat sensitivities, which vary with the type of organism and the environment to which they are accustomed. For example, bacterial spores are more resistant than the vegetative form of the bacteria. In a closed container like autoclave, where the volume remains same, increase in pressure raises the temperature as well. If items are exposed long enough to steam at a specified temperature and pressure, they become sterile.

Two types of autoclave indicator includes chemical indicators system, which undergoes a colour change on exposure to sterilizing temperatures, and biological indicators, such as heat-resistant bacterial spores (*e.g.*, *Bacillus stearothermophilus*). Spores of thermophilic aerobes and anaerobes are the most resistant forms of life to moist heat known. Virus particles are much less tolerant to steam sterilization than are spores.

Recognized minimum exposure periods for sterilization of wrapped healthcare supplies are 30 minutes at 121° C (250° F) in a gravity displacement sterilizer or 4 minutes at 132° C (270° F) in a prevacuum sterilizer. Steam gives up its heat to materials to be sterilized by the process of condensation, and it is able to penetrate porous substances more rapidly than dry heat.

Sterilization failure may occur if packs are wrapped too tightly or are improperly loaded in the autoclave or gas sterilizer container. Instrument packs should be positioned vertically (*i.e.*, on edge) and longitudinally in an autoclave. Heavy packs should be placed at the periphery, where steam enters the chamber. A small amount of air space is allowed between the packs to facilitate the flow of steam (1 to 2 inches between the packs and away from the surrounding walls). Linen packs are loaded so that the fabric layers are oriented vertically (*i.e.*, on edge). These packs are not stacked because the increased thickness reduces penetration of the steam. Close supervision and exact standards for preparing, packaging and loading of instruments are necessary for effective steam and gas sterilization. Sterilization indicators should be used.

Filtration

Sterilization by filtration is used for air supply to surgery rooms (laminar flow ventilation), in industrial preparation of medications, and for small volumes of solutions in practice settings. For the sterilization of serum, antibiotic solutions, carbohydrate solutions and media that are heat labile, filtration is used in which microbes are removed from liquids by means of filters with very small pores that trap bacteria. In order to remove bacteria, the membrane pore size must be smaller than the bacteria and uniform throughout.

Chemical (Gas) Sterilization

Ethylene Oxide (ETO)

ETO is a flammable, explosive, gas that kills micro-organisms by altering their deoxyribonucleic acid (DNA) through alkylation and it is effective against vegetative bacteria, fungi, viruses and spores. It is the most commonly used agent in chemical sterilization. Because it is a gas, it rapidly penetrates packaging and items to be sterilized at temperatures tolerated by almost all materials. However, its use is limited by the size of the equipment, the time requirement, and concerns about toxicity. It is recommended for equipment that cannot withstand the extreme temperature and pressures of steam sterilization (*i.e.*, endoscopes, cameras, plastics, and power cables).

Sterilization by ethylene oxide is influenced by gas concentration (450-1200 mg/l), temperature 120°-140°F (49°-60°C), humidity (20–80 per cent) (water molecules carry ETO to reactive sites), and exposure time (1-6 hours). The time required for sterilization depends on the concentration of ETO, humidity level, temperature, density and type of materials to be sterilized. However, the main disadvantages associated with ETO are lengthy cycle time, the cost and its potential hazards to the patient and hospital personnel.

After sterilization by ETO, materials must be aerated to allow dissipation of the absorbed chemical, because residual ethylene oxide can damage tissues. ETO is absorbed by many materials. The specific aeration time necessary for surgical items depends on many variables, including the composition and size of the item, its preparation and packaging, the type of ETO sterilizer used, and the type of aerator. The manufacturer's guidelines should be followed, but generally aeration in a well-ventilated area for a minimum of 7 days, or 12-18 hours in an aerator, is sufficient. Items should be clean and dry before ETO sterilization, moisture and organic material bond with ETO and leave a toxic residue. Exposure to ethylene oxide can cause skin and mucous membrane irritation, nausea, vomiting, headache, cognitive impairment, sensory loss, reproductive failure and increased incidence of chromosomal abnormalities. The Environmental Protection Agency (EPA) has classified ETO as a Group B1, probable human carcinogen.

Plasma Sterilization

Plasma sterilization is a low-temperature sterilization technique that has become the method of choice for sterilizing heat-sensitive items. Conventional sterilization techniques (*e.g.*, autoclaves, ovens, chemicals like ETO) rely on irreversible metabolic inactivation or on breakdown of vital structural components of the micro-organism. Plasma sterilization operates differently because it uses ultraviolet (UV) photons and radicals. An advantage of the plasma method is the possibility of sterilizing at relatively low temperatures (50°C), preserving the integrity of polymer-based instruments, which cannot be subjected to sterilization by autoclaves or ovens. Furthermore, plasma sterilization is safe, both for the operator and the patient, in contrast to ETO. Vapour phase hydrogen peroxide sterilization is a form of plasma sterilization that uses hydrogen peroxide to process instruments quickly and efficiently.

Instruments can be sterilized at low temperatures (*i.e.*, below 122° F [50°C]) and short time intervals (*i.e.*, 45 minutes), and they are immediately available because aeration is not required.

Gas plasma is suitable for heat- and moisture-sensitive instruments (rigid endoscopy lenses and instrument sets, objective lenses for microscopes, nonfabric tourniquets, medication vials, aluminum, brass, silicone, teflon, latex, ethyl vinyl acetate, polycarbonate, polyethylene (high density and low density), polyolefin, polyurethane, polypropylene, polyvinyl chloride (PVC), and polymethyl-methacrylate, insulated electrosurgery and cautery instruments, and metal instruments). The sharpness of the delicate microsurgical instruments remains unchanged.

Gas plasma is unsuitable for flexible endoscopes, some plastics, liquids, and items derived from plant fibers (paper products, linens, gauze sponges, wood products including paper, Q-tip applicators, cast padding, gloves and single-use items), because these materials absorb hydrogen peroxide and inhibit sterilization. Items that cannot be disassembled or completely dried, items with copper or silver solder or that use bisphenole epoxy, very long narrow lumens, lumens closed at one end, folded plastic bags, and sheeting are unsuitable for sterilization by gas plasma. An important shortcoming of plasma sterilization is its dependence on the actual "thickness" of the micro-organisms to be inactivated because UV photons need to reach the DNA. Any material covering the micro-organisms (*e.g.*, packaging) will slow down the process.

Ionizing Radiation

Sterilization by radiation is used in the industrial preparation of surgical materials that are sensitive to heat or chemical agents. Items commonly sterilized with ionizing radiation include suture materials, sponges, disposable items (*i.e.*, gowns, drapes and table covers), powders and petroleum goods. Re-sterilization by other means may not be possible for pre-packaged sterilized items that have been opened but not used because an alternate technique could damage the item and create a health hazard.

Cold Chemical Sterilization

Chemicals used for sterilization must be noncorrosive to the items being sterilized. Glutaraldehyde is a saturated dialdehyde that has gained wide acceptance as a high-level disinfectant and chemical sterilant. The biocidal activity of glutaraldehyde results from its alkylation of sulfhydryl, hydroxyl, carboxyl and amino groups of micro-organisms, which alters RNA, DNA and protein synthesis. Aqueous solutions of glutaraldehyde are acidic and generally in this state are not sporicidal. Only when the solution is "activated" (made alkaline) by use of alkalinating agents to pH 7.5–8.5 does the solution become sporicidal. It is noncorrosive to metals, rubbers and plastics, and provides a means of sterilizing delicate lensed instruments (*i.e.*, endoscopes, cystoscopes and bronchoscopes). Most equipment that are safe for immersion in water are safe for immersion in 2 per cent glutaraldehyde. For the high level disinfection of endoscopes, a 2 per cent glutaraldehyde solution without surfactant is recommended. Items for sterilization should be clean and dry; organic matter (*e.g.*, blood, saliva) may prevent penetration of crevices or joints. Residual water causes chemical dilution. Complex instruments should be disassembled before immersion. After the appropriate immersion period, instruments should be rinsed thoroughly with sterile water and dried with sterile towels to prevent damaging the patients' tissues.

The major problems associated with glutaraldehyde are skin irritation or dermatitis, mucous membrane irritation (eye, nose, mouth), or pulmonary symptoms, epistaxis, allergic contact dermatitis, asthma and rhinitis in healthcare workers exposed to glutaraldehyde. Failure to rinse disinfected equipment thoroughly, leaving residual glutaraldehyde on the endoscope, has led to serious conditions, including chemical colitis, pancreatitis and mucosal damage in human patients.

4

Sutures and Suturing Techniques

M.M.S. Zama

Suture, a Latin word '*Sutura*' means 'seam', a line formed by sewing together 2 pieces of any matter. In other words, it is the surgical uniting of 2 surfaces by means of stitches. However, it is also referred to a material/surgical thread that is used to ligate off the vessels or any hollow organ or keeping the organs or tissues in place. There is another term 'Suturing' which is the temporary anatomical reconstruction (reduction, alignment and fixation) of severed ends of soft tissue by appropriate suture material. Surgical thread that is used to tie off the blood vessels or any hollow structure is ligature.

Ambriose Pare (1556) first applied suturing thread on blood vessels and Joseph Lister (1876) invented the chromatization of catgut to delay its absorption. Currently, a number of suture materials are available and selection of appropriate suture material is determined by its characteristics (physical and biological properties), knowledge of local conditions and healing rate of the wound, rather than on training, experience and preference of the surgeon. None of the currently available suture materials possess all the ideal characteristics, however, many have excellent characteristics.

Properties of an Ideal Suture

☆ Possess tensile strength corresponding to the wound where it is applied

☆ Easy to handle with good knot security

☆ Non-electrolytic, non-capillary, non-allergenic and non-carcinogenic

☆ Stimulate minimal tissue reaction

☆ Does not predispose to oedematous inflammation

☆ Bio-inert and passes through the tissues without any friction

☆ Inexpensive, easily available and easy to sterilize without alteration

Classification

Sutures are generally classified as absorbable or non-absorbable sutures based on their rate of degradation and loss of tensile strength. Suture materials that retain tensile strength for longer than 60 days are classified as non-absorbable while those materials which lose their tensile strength within that period are classified as absorbable. Further, sutures may also be classified based on the source (natural or synthetic) or on thickness (thickest: 6 and superfine: 15-0).

Natural Absorbable Suture Materials

Catgut (Surgical Gut/Surgigut)

Catgut is prepared either from the submucosa of sheep small intestine or serosal layer of cattle small intestine and is essentially composed of formaldehyde treated collagen. It is a capillary multifilament and is ground precisely in order to achieve a monofilament character. Being collagenous in nature, it stimulates a significant foreign body reaction at the site of implantation. Surgical gut is available in plain and chromic forms. Treatment with chromic salts increases its tensile strength and resistance to digestion, and also decreases tissue reactivity. Depending on the site of implantation, its rate of absorption and loss of tensile strength varies. Premature absorption occurs in infected environments, gastric secretions and highly vascularized tissues. Surgical catgut absorption occurs by two fold mechanism, primarily by macrophages. First, acid hydrolytic and collagenolytic activity cleave molecular bonds followed by digestion and absorption through proteolytic enzymes. It can be sterilized by ionizing radiation or by ethylene oxide. Sterilization by ethylene oxide prolongs its absorption time.

Catgut generally exhibits good handling characteristics but poor knot security, when wet. Its disadvantages are intense inflammatory reaction, variability in loss of tensile strength, its capillarity and occasional sensitivity reaction, especially in cats.

Collagen

Collagen, a multifilament suture material is obtained by processing of bovine flexor tendon with formaldehyde or chromic salts or both. Its advantages over catgut are its non-septic source and simplicity in processing. Its rate and method of absorption resemble to those of catgut. These sutures are almost exclusively used for ophthalmic surgery.

Kangaroo Tendon

It is obtained from tail of Kangaroo and has very high tensile strength. It is used at high tension sites and where suture is required for very long time *e.g.*, bovine capsule suturing.

Fascia Lata

It is obtained from bovine fascia lata and is used for additional support to the fascial layers.

Synthetic Absorbable Suture Materials

Polyglycolic Acid (Dexon)

Polyglycolic acid (PGA) is a braided multifilament, glycolic acid polymer, which gets absorbed by hydrolysis (esterases) and not by phagocytosis. Alkaline conditions hasten its hydrolysis hence its use is not recommended in the urinary bladder. It has superior tensile strength compared to surgical gut, but it loses its strength more rapidly. In acute stages of infection, there is marked reaction against the PGA than at later stages. It tends to drag through the tissues, cuts friable tissues and has relatively poor knot security.

Polyglactin 910 (Vicryl)

It is the braided multifilament, synthetic absorbable suture material and is composed of glycolic acid and lactic acids in the ratio of 9:1. Compared to PGA, it is more hydrophobic and resistant to hydrolysis. Its absorption occurs by same mechanism as that of PGA and also has similar pattern of loss of tensile strength as that of PGA. Polyglactin has an excellent size-to-strength ratio, is relatively easy to handle, stable in contaminated wounds and elicits minimal tissue reaction.

Polydiaxanone

It is a monofilament suture material composed of polymer of paradiaxanone and is more flexible than PGA and polyglactin 910. It incites little tissue reaction. Polydiaxanone is absorbed by hydrolysis similar to that of PGA/polyglactin.

Non-absorbable Suture Materials

Silk

It is obtained from the silk worm cocoons and is available as braided multifilament. Capillary action can be reduced by treating it with oil, wax or silicone. It is readily available, inexpensive and easy to sterilize. Silk has excellent handling characteristics; however, weaker in terms of strength and knot security. Other disadvantages of silk include tissue reactions, potential to produce ulcerations if protrudes into the lumen, and act as nidus for calculi formation in the lumen of urinary bladder or gall bladder. Its use should also be avoided in infected wounds as the interstices between its fibers allow serum and blood to penetrate leading to bacterial growth.

Cotton

It is readily available and inexpensive multifilament suture material that can be autoclaved. In contrast to silk its tensile strength and knot security increases *in vivo*. Its disadvantages include capillarity, tissue reactivity, inferior handling ability (electrostatic property) and ability to potentiate infection.

Nylon

It is available as both monofilament as well as multifilament suture material. It is biologically inert and produces minimal tissue reaction. It has an intermediate tensile strength. It can be used in infected tissues as reaction to nylon in such tissues is very less. It is not recommended to use nylon in serous or synovial cavities as sharp ends may incite tissue reaction. The main disadvantage of nylon includes poor handling characteristics and knot security. It is generally being called to possess 'Memory' which is the tendency to revert back to the original configuration. To prevent that it is generally being applied by 'surgeons reinforced knot or nylon knot'.

Polypropylene

It is a polymer of propylene and is available as monofilament suture. It possesses relatively low tensile strength but high knot security, and is ductile and tough. Its knot security is superior to all other monofilament nonmetallic suture materials. It retains its strength on implantation in tissue as it is not weakened by tissue enzymes. It is the least thrombogenic suture material available and is frequently used in vascular surgeries. Due to its high flexibility it is used for closing tissues with great elongation capability (cardiac muscle and skin). Its disadvantage is slippery handling and tying characteristics.

Stainless Steel

It is the only metallic suture that is currently being used. It is available as monofilament or twisted multifilament, and is biologically inert, non-capillary (monofilament), and can be sterilized by autoclaving. Stainless steel possesses highest knot security of all the suture materials available with no inflammatory reaction. Monofilament form does not support infection and can be used in infected wounds. Its disadvantages include tendency to cut through the tissues, poor handling characteristics and tendency to break on repeated bending.

Suture Techniques

Significance of Suture Patterns

☆ Impact on the apposition of tissues

☆ Plays a large role in wound healing

☆ Specific patterns can be used to accurately appose tissues, distribute wound tension, invert suture lines, and approximate the ends of tendons

There are number of suture patterns that have been described for animal use and have been categorized into different groups according to the following factors:

☆ Tendency to overcome tension- like tension sutures

☆ Anatomical area of application- like skin sutures, tendon sutures, etc

☆ Fashion in which applied like- interrupted or continuous

☆ Ability to promote apposition, inversion or eversion of the tissue margins

Some of the important suture patterns which are commonly used at field level are given below:

Name of Pattern	Wound Edge	Consideration	Possible Indications
Simple interrupted	Apposition	Interrupted	Skin, subcutaneous tissue, fascia, nerve, blood vessels
Intradermal/subcuticular	Apposition	Interrupted/ continuous	Subcutaneous tissue
Cruciate/crossMattress	Apposition	Interrupted	Skin, stump of tail, digits
Horizontal mattress	Apposition/everted	interrupted	Skin, subcutaneous tissue
Vertical mattress	Apposition/eversion	Interrupted	Skin, subcutaneous tissue, fascia
Far-near-near-far	Apposition	Interrupted	Skin, subcutaneous tissue, fascia
Far-far-near-near	Apposition	Interrupted	Skin, subcutaneous tissue, fascia
Overlapping/Vest overpant	Overlapping	Sustain maximum tension	Ventral or abdominal hernias
Simple continuous	Apposition	Continuous	Subcutaneous tissue, fascia, muscles, blood vessels
Running suture	Apposition	Continuous	Peritoneum, thin muscle layer, loose connective tissue
Lock stitch/ford	Apposition	Continuous	Diaphragm, interlocking muscle layers
Lambert	Inversion	Interrupted/ continuous	Hollow organs like stomach, uterus, urinary bladder
Halstead	Inversion	Interrupted	Hollow organs like stomach, uterus, urinary bladder
Jobert	Inversion	Interrupted/ continuous	Hollow organs like stomach, uterus, urinary bladder
Cushing	Inversion	Interrupted/ continuous	Hollow organs like stomach, uterus, urinary bladder
Connell	Inversion	Interrupted/ continuous	Hollow organs like stomach, uterus, urinary bladder
Locking loop/ Modified Kessler	Apposition	Interrupted	Tendon
Intraneural	Apposition	Interrupted	Nerves

Tissue	Consideration	Suture Pattern	Material	Size
1. Skin	No capillary action, allows drainage	Simple interrupted, horizontal mattress	Monofilament nylon, silk, stainless steel	1-0 to 3-0 (S.A) 1 to 2 (L.A)
2. Subcutaneous tissue/fascia	Absorbable suture material	Subcuticular, simple interrupted, lock stitch, vertical mattress	PGA, polyglactin, polydiaxanone, catgut, collagen	1-0 to 3-0 (S.A) 1 to 2-0 (L.A)
3. Peritoneum, Pleura	Least tissue reaction, absorbable, air and water tight	Running or simple continous	PGA, polyglactin, catgut	2-0 to 3-0 (S.A) 1-0 to 1 (L.A)
4. Hollow organs (Except urinary tract)	No capillary action, water tight and absorbable	Inverted sutures	PGA, poly-glactin, catgut, polydiaxanone	3-0 to 4-0 (S.A) 1-0 to 1 (L.A)
5. Urinary tract	Absorbable and water tight	Inverted or lock stitch	Catgut, PGA, polyglactin, polydiaxanone	3-0 to 4-0 (S.A) 2-0 to 1-0 (L.A)
6. Blood vessels	Least thrombo-genic, water tight and least tissue reaction	Simple continuous or simple interrupted	For suturing (polypropylene, nylon, silk) and for ligation (PGA, plain catgut, silk)	4-0 to 7-0 (S.A) 4-0 to 2-0 (L.A)
7. Nerves	Least tissue	Simple reaction	Nylon, poly-propylene	4-0 to 7-0
8. Tendon or ligament	Bear tension and have strength for long time	Bunnel Mayer, vertical mattress, cross mattress	Stainless steel, nylon, poly-diaxanone	3-0 to 0 (S.A) 2-3 (L.A)

SA: Small Animals and LA: Large Animals.

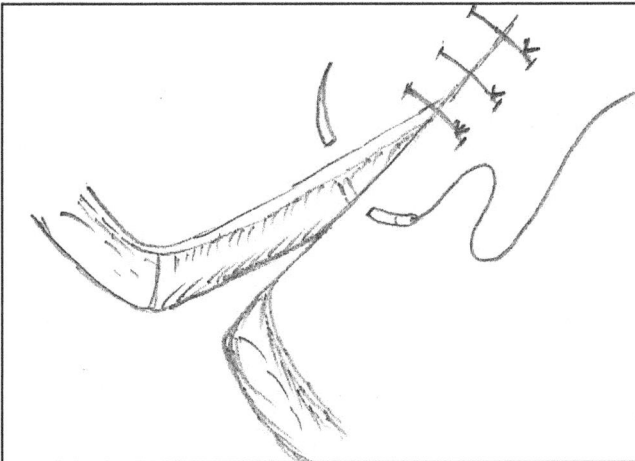

Figure 4.1: Simple Interrupted Suture

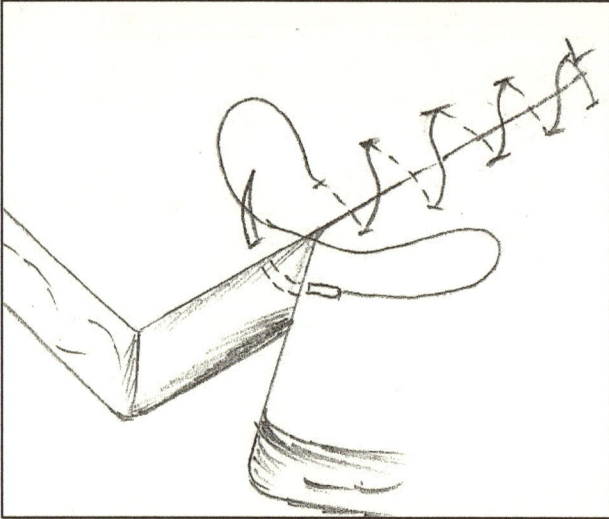

Figure 4.2: Simple Continuous Suture

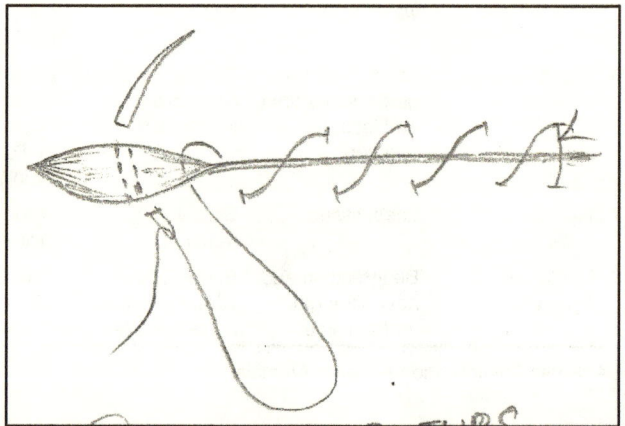

Figure 4.3: Running Suture

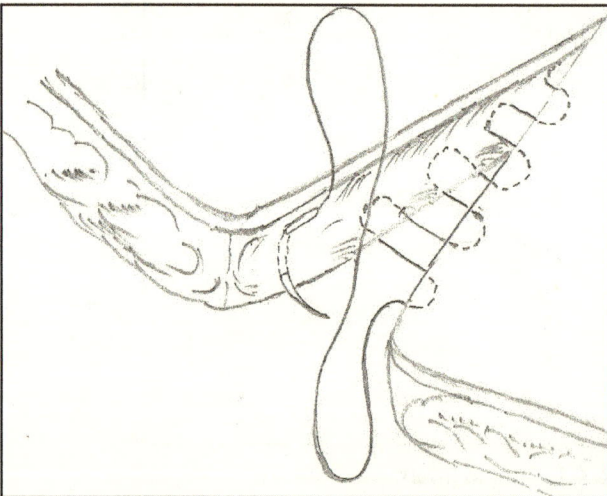

Figure 4.4: Subcutaneous Suture

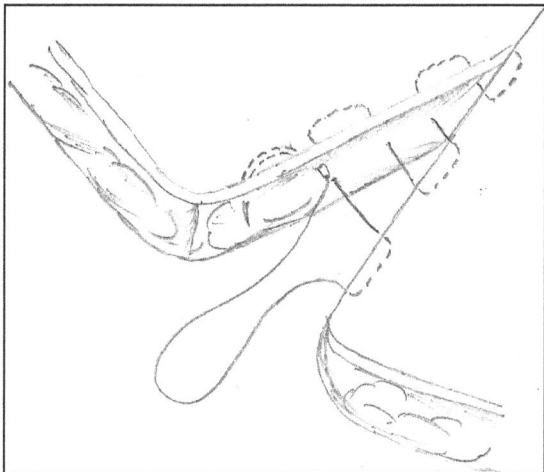

Figure 4.5: Sub-cuticular Suture

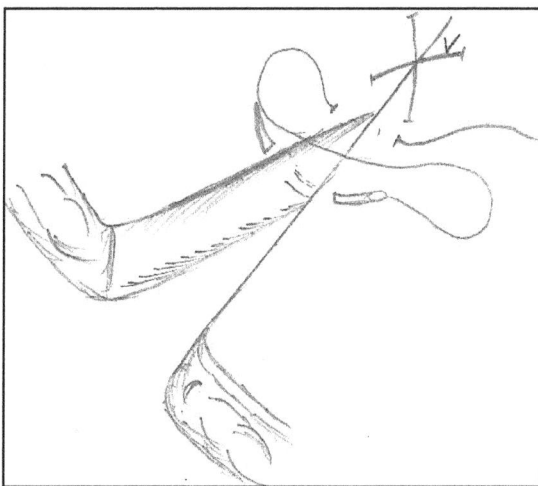

Figure 4.6: Cruciate Suture

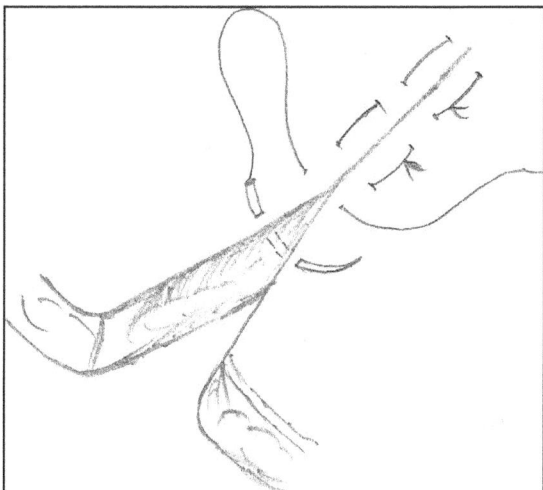

Figure 4.7: Horizontal Mattress Suture

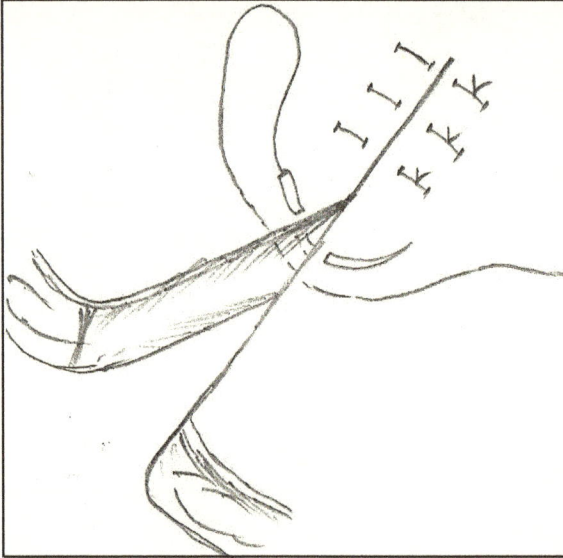

Figure 4.8: Vertical Mattress Suture

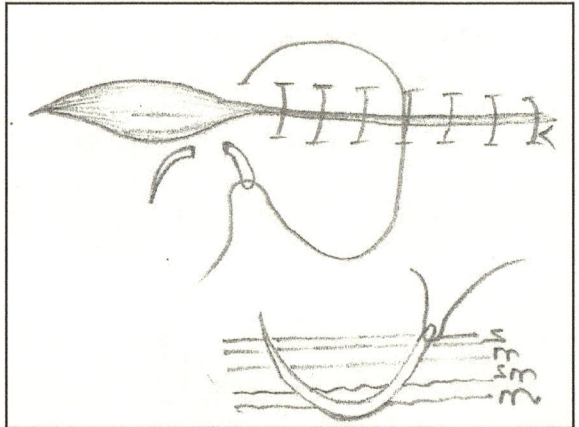

Figure 4.9: Connel Suture

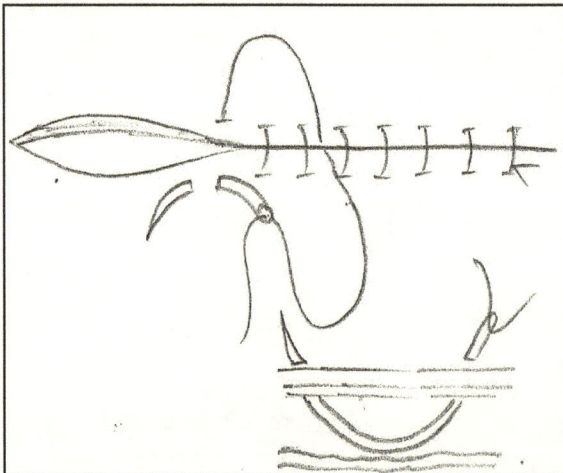

Figure 4.10: Cushing Suture

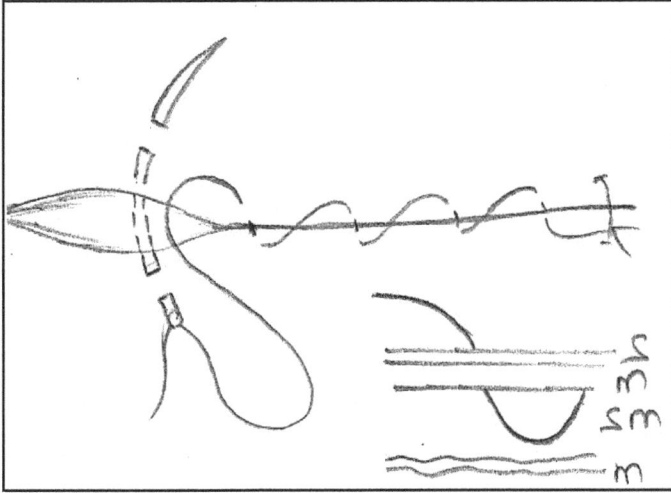

Figure 4.11:
Lambert Suture

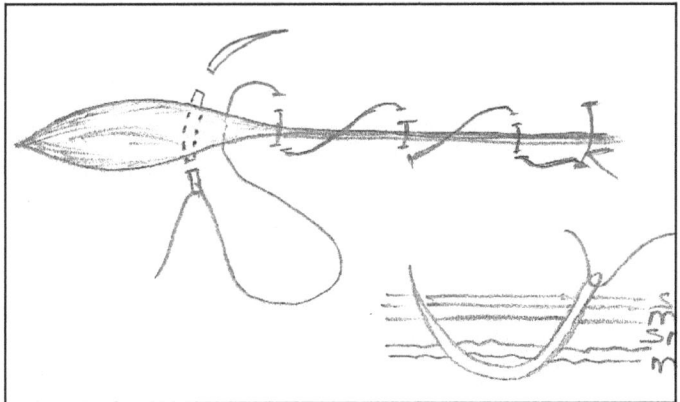

Figure 4.12:
Jobert Suture

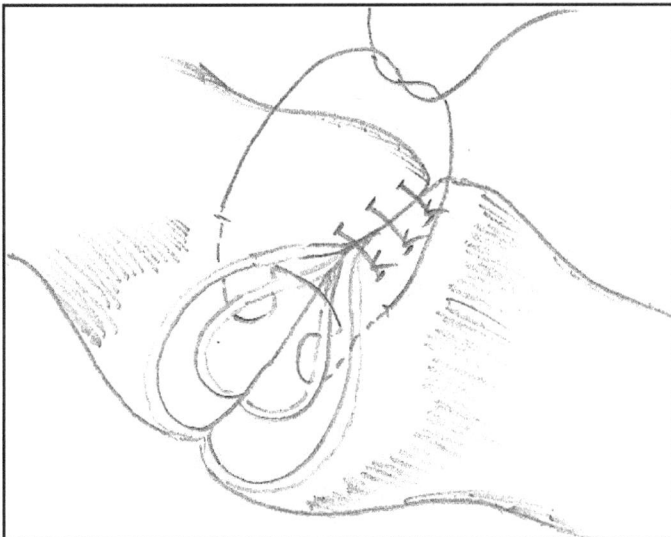

Figure 4.13:
Gambee Suture

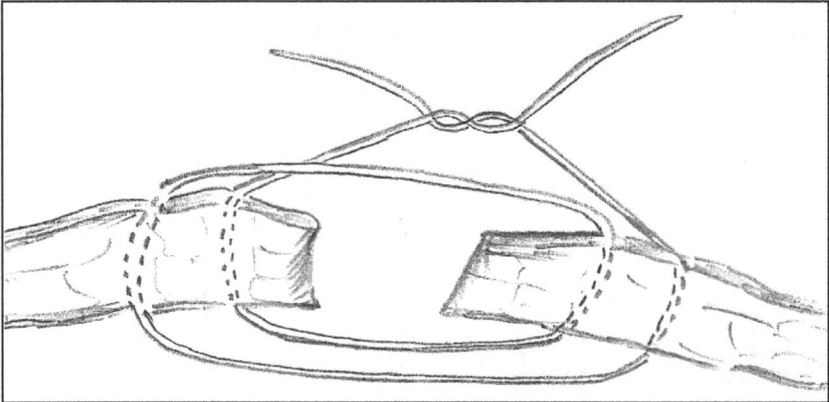

Figure 4.14: Far-Far-Near-Near Suture

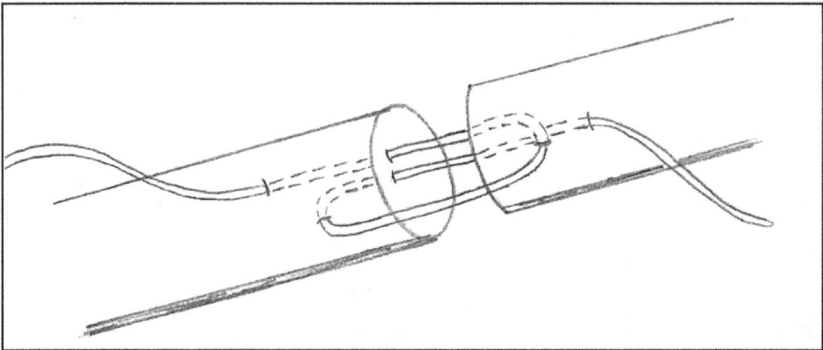

Figure 4.15: Far-Near-Near-Far Suture

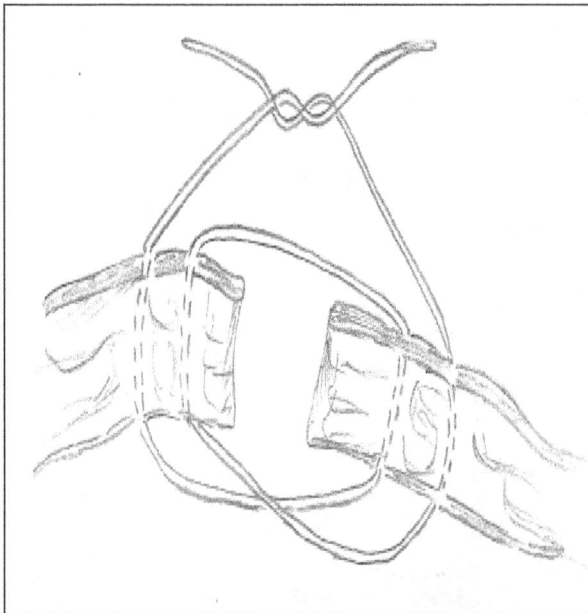

Figure 4.16: Far-Near-Near-Far Suture

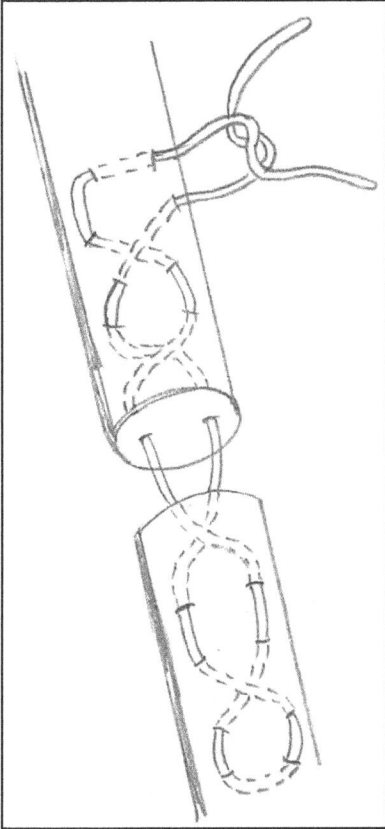

Figure 4.17: Bunnel Suture

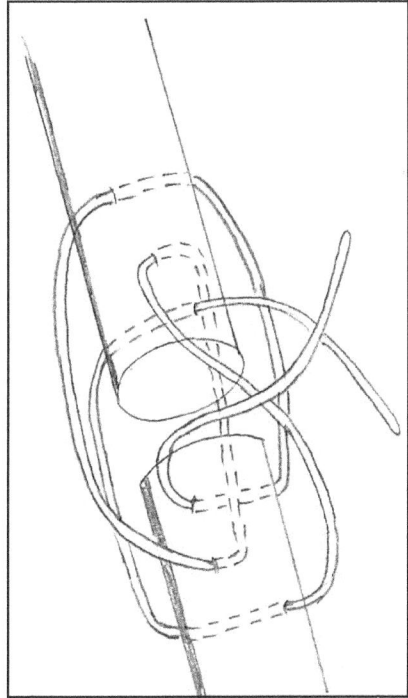

Figure 4.18: Tree Loop Pulley

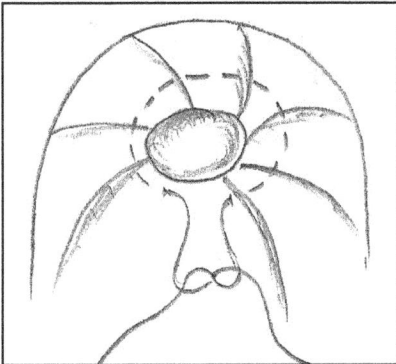

Figure 4.19: Purse String Suture

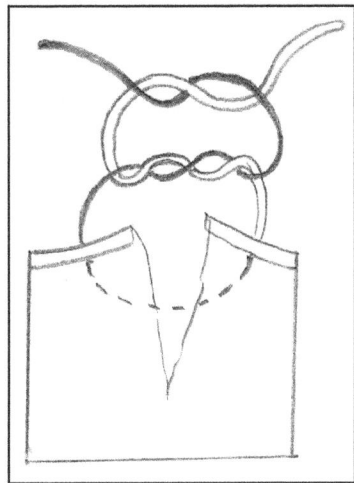

Figure 4.20: Surgeon's Knot

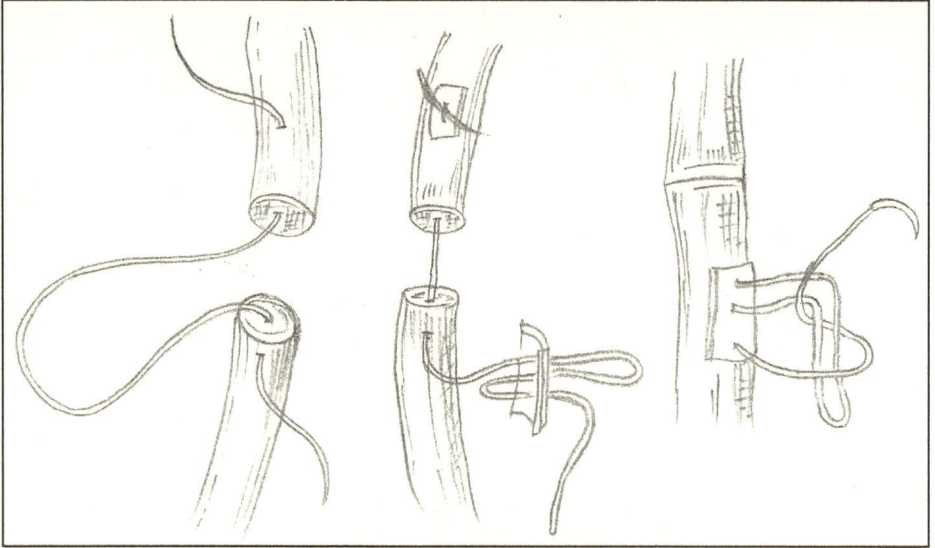

Figure 4.21: Intraneural Suture

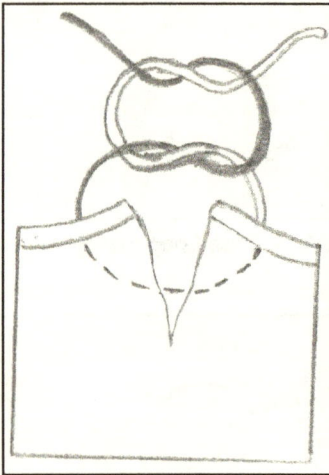

Figure 4.22(a):
Square Knot

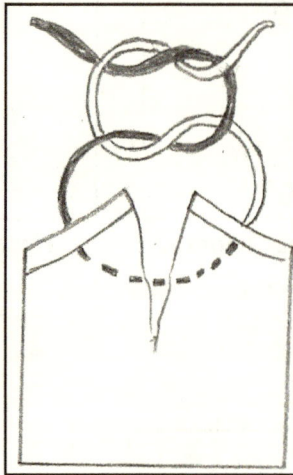

Figure 4.22(b):
Granny Knot

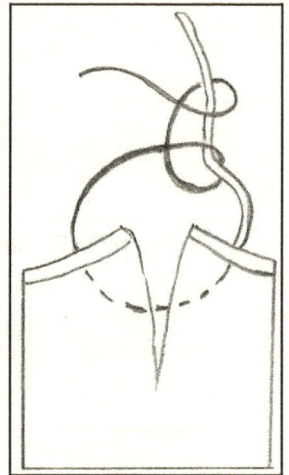

Figure 4.22(c):
Half Hitch Knot

5

Management of Wounds

A.M. Pawde

Wound is a separation or discontinuity of skin' mucous membrane or tissue surface caused by physical, chemical or biological insult. Wound healing is restoration of this continuity.

Type of Wounds

- ☆ **Incised:** caused by sharp object
- ☆ **Lacerated:** tearing of tissue with peculiar jagged, irregular border
- ☆ **Penetrating**: caused by long pointed objects may lead to communication with body cavities and deep seated infections
- ☆ **Gunshot wounds:** caused by firearms, intensity depends on the velocity of bullets may lead to incised, lacerated or contused wound
- ☆ **Poisoned wounds:** caused by poisons or toxins
- ☆ **Bite wounds:** caused by bites of dogs, wild animals, snakes or birds
- ☆ **Virulent wounds:** caused by virus or bacteria, lead to formation of pustules or vesicles
- ☆ **Ulcerative wounds:** caused by surface evacuated due to slough of necrotic debris *e.g.,* ischemic necrosis
- ☆ **Erosive wounds:** necrotic areas confined only to epidermis
- ☆ **Punctured wounds:** caused by blunt or sharp objects, they are deep and invite anaerobes
- ☆ **Abrasions:** denuded areas of skin and mucous membrane

☆ **Contusions or bruises:** no discontinuity in skin but damage to muscles, tendon, bones and nerves.

General Management of Wounds

Healing is a natural and inherent biological process and body keeps this process on priority than other functions. Clinician acts as a positive catalyst in accelerating the wound healing process in a shortest time with minimal scar and deformity and without complication. On the basis of injury causing agent, time elapsed and the condition of the surroundings, the wounds are classified as: (i) clean, (ii) contaminated, (iii) septic or infected, and (iv) accidental or traumatic wounds.

Clean or Aseptic (Surgical) Wounds

In spite of taking all possible aseptic measures at the surgical site (clipping hair, washing with detergent and surgical scrub several times, finally with 1 per cent povidone iodine and the draping at the site) and surgical instruments, no open wound is absolutely aseptic and every wound has some infection. In horses, camels, sheep, goats and calves tetanus prophylaxis is mandatory. Wound exposure time should be minimum, tissue not allowed to be desiccated by heat, rough handling of tissue to be avoided and haemorrhage must be kept minimum. The wound is mopped to keep it dry, blood clots removed, drain placed and skin sutures applied using monofilament suture with a fine swaged needle. To reduce infection, suturing of highly contaminated wound must be avoided, and antibiotic has to be administered in bacterial infection. It is, however, said that antibiotic cover for a surgical wound is a poor substitute for a good surgical technique. Nevertheless, prophylactic (antibiotic umbrella) or therapeutic use of antibiotic systemically is more beneficial than topical wound dressing. Use of fly repellant is inevitable in summer months. A sutured wound heals within 7-14 days if the wound is under dressing, immobilized and the part is at rest. Sutures are to be removed after 10th post-operative day on assessing the wound status, if healing is not complete then alternate suture/stitch can be removed. Even after complete removal of stitches the wound needs dressing for at least 3=4 days to heal the "suture needle pricks" (suture bites). Animal has to be cared for another 15 days; it may scratch, rub or bite the wound and increase the risk of infection and wound dehiscence.

Contaminated and Septic Wound

In a fresh wound up to 6 hours in which the tissue reaction has not yet established, antibiotic has to be started immediately, infection sets in only if there is tissue ischemia. A contaminated wound should be properly taken care:

☆ Identify the microbes

☆ Foreign materials inside the wound should be removed

☆ Wound irrigated with normal saline solution

☆ An antiseptic solution is poured with the help of syringe jet first with 0.1 per cent chlorinated water and 2 per cent hydrogen peroxide

☆ Once again wash with the chlorinated water and finally 1 per cent tamed povidone iodine is applied

☆ Topical debridement may be achieved with 2.5 per cent NaCl or magnesium sulphate-glycerine paste

☆ Linen (shroud and drapes) may be applied over the wound to prevent contamination

☆ A fenestrated tube as a drain is placed to favour drainage of the exudate

Infected Wound

The wound more than 6-8 hours after injury with inflammatory reaction in tissue becomes infected. It may be treated as an open wound. Deep penetrating wound harbour anaerobic infection. These wounds are seldom sutured, unless infection is checked. Wound is lavaged with 0.5 per cent sodium hypochlorite in small animals and 0.5 per cent potassium permanganate solution in large animals. Systemic (preferred) antibiotics have to be started. Drain tube may be placed to favour drainage of pus, serum or exudate etc. The tube is removed after 5 days.

On assessing the status of wounds, dressing has to be undertaken whether antiseptic, maggoticide or escharotic. The hollow of the wound has to be filled with cream or ointment and finally covered with sterile gauze; likewise wound dressing has has to be changed after every 24 hours for 7-9 days. If there is an oedema or accumulation of pus, then a counter stab incision should be given on the dependent part to facilitate drainage of the exudate.

On cessation of exudation from the wound it may be dressed on alternate days, thereafter biweekly and later on weekly once. Luke warm flushing in chronic wounds is helpful. Foreign bodies if any have to be removed. Suturing of wound may be done with monofilament synthetic non-absorbable material after infection is controlled.

Accidental Traumatic Wounds

Haemorrhage has to be checked to avoid shock. Shock if present has to be treated by replenishing the fluid loss and providing warmth to the patient. Septicaemia should be prevented by administration of proper antibiotics. Tetanus toxoid must be given in horses, camels, sheep, goats and calves. The wound should be flushed with chilled normal saline, which will help in washing away the dirt. The principles of treatment approach in such cases might be (i) cleansing, (ii) exicision, (iii) debridement, and (iv) delayed primary closure. A course of antibiotic must be given for at least 10 days.

Complications of Wound Healing

☆ Haemorrhage

☆ Wound dehiscence

☆ Traumatic neuralgia

☆ Traumatic fever and septicemia

☆ Traumatic emphysema

☆ Tetanus

☆ Haematoma

☆ Sinus

☆ Fistula

☆ Cellulitis

☆ Exuberant granulation tissue

Topical Wound Medication

A topical preparation should be eco-friendly, earlier agents were proven destroyers of WBCs and other cellular elements. Phenyl, disinfectant used for mopping the floor, is sometimes used by quacks to kill maggots, diesel to flush otorrhoea, deltamethrin or malathion as maggoticide. The use of these drugs is inhuman as they may cause pain to the animal, delay healing of wounds and it is dangerous to human health if meat and milk of such animals are consumed. Therefore, mild antiseptic solutions should be used. Hypertonic saline (2.5 per cent NaCl) has cleansing as well as antibacterial effect but it irritates tissue and cause negative chemotaxis. Povidone iodine (0.1-1 per cent) has higher concentration of free iodine, which has high bactericidal activity, however, at higher concentration (10 per cent) it inhibits WBCs migration, fibroblastic and tissue cellularity. Chlorhexidine 0.05 per cent is more effective as sporicide, very effective in dirty wounds, especially with clostridial spores. Sodium hypochlorite 0.5 per cent solution release chlorine and oxygen in tissues, kills bacteria and liquefies tissues. Ointment of bacitracin, neomycin and polymyxin as well as nitrofurazone and gentamicin solution were widely used for wound care in veterinary practice. Oxoferrin (Tetrachlor decpoxide) similar to hydrogen peroxide helps in bringing more of haemoglobin toward wound and thereby hastening wound healing, provided it is used alone. Besides this, for large wounds, topical anabolic steroids with neomycin ointment (Clostagen, Elder Co.) is very effective. Chemical debridement agents or escharotics like copper sulphate, silver nitrate, potassium permanganate granules have some disadvantages like irritation, which provokes the animal for mutilation, however, use of collagenase enzyme (Salutyl; Elder) as an ointment helps in overcoming this problem.

Honey contains 40 per cent glucose and is rich in essential amino acids and vitamins, which are useful for treatment of burns and sores. Similarly the butter oil preparations in combination with olive oil were also used for cracked teats, but they are known to reduce wound epithelization.

Herbal drugs like *Curcuma longa, Eriolaenia quinquelocularis, Moringa pterygospermia, Adhatoda vasica, Phyllanthus niruri, Allium sativum, Helianthus armous, Anona squamosa, Adonsonia digitala/vulgaris, Calendula officinalis, Achrynthes asperia, Eclipta alba, Tridex procumbens* etc. have been claimed to be potent accelerators of wound healing.

Biological wound dressings like potato peel, banana leaf, bovine tracheal cartilage powder, liver spleen powder and amnion have been also used as promoters of wound healing.

Bandaging

The primary contact layers of bandage are of two types (a) adherent, and (b) non adherent. These bandages must be sterile as they come in direct contact with wound surface.

Adherent Bandages

   ☆ *Dry to dry:* A dry bandage is applied in lightly oozing wound; while removing or changing the dressing, normal saline is poured to detach adhered bandage

   ☆ *Wet to dry:* Bandage soaked in normal saline are applied and later on water soluble antibiotics are sprinkled

   ☆ *Wet to wet:* Bandages mostly dry, hygroscopic agent is used to liquefy the thick exudate.

Non Adherent Bandages

   ☆ Petrolatum impregnated squared gauze

   ☆ Secondary layer

   ☆ Tertiary layer

Abscess

An abscess is an abnormal cavity containing pus, which is lined by pyogenic membrane.

Types

   ☆ *Acute (hot) abscess:* in this the inflammatory symptoms are quite active

   ☆ *Chronic (cold) abscess:* in this the inflammatory symptoms are less active, the pus may become partly inspissated or liquefied

   ☆ *Superficial abscess:* it is situated superficially

   ☆ *Deep abscess:* an abscess that is deep seated

   ☆ *Embolic abscess:* developing from a septic embolus

   ☆ *Pyaemic or metastatic abscess:* a number of abscess developing in different parts of the body.

Differential Diagnosis

An abscess should be differentiated from a cyst, a haematoma, a synovial distension or an abdominal hernia. A cyst develops slowly and fluctuates uniformly. A haematoma (containing coagulated blood and stream) has a doughy consistency and may crepitate on palpation. It is not painful and does not point like an abscess. A distended synovial sheath is recognized by its location and by careful palpation. An abdominal hernia can be differentiated by the presence of hernia ring.

Confirmatory diagnosis can be made by exploratory puncture, which helps to find out the nature of contents.

Treatment

Fomentation and/or application of blisters (Bin iodide of mercury) are advised to bring about early maturation of the abscess. However, abscess situated close to a joint or peritoneum may have to be opened before fully mature, to avoid the chances of rupture into the joint or peritoneal cavity. After preparation of the site aseptically, an opening is made at the level of pointing with the help of BP blade No. 15. If the abscess is not pointing at the dependent portion, it is sometimes necessary to make another opening in the dependent part to provide drainage. This is called "counter-opening". After opening the abscess, the abscess cavity should be irrigated with hypertonic saline, and then it is packed with the tincture iodine dipped gauze. Gauze pack is removed after 24 hr and then the abscess cavity is irrigated with a mild antiseptic lotion. From 2nd day onwards, the abscess cavity is packed with magnesium sulphate-glycerine paste, which greatly favours drainage and absorption of exudates. Bismuth iodine paraffin paste (BIPP) is a conventional antiseptic dressing used. It contains bismuth subnitras (1 parts) and iodoform (2 parts) mixed in liquid paraffin to form a paste of desired consistency.

Factor Affecting Wound Healing

Local Factors

☆ Surgical technique
☆ Tissue vascularity
☆ Mechanical stress
☆ Movement
☆ Extent of wound surface
☆ Haemorrhage
☆ Foreign bodies
☆ Oedema and dehydration
☆ Local irradiation
☆ Suture material and technique
☆ Wound infection
☆ Topical application

Systemic Factors

☆ Age
☆ Obesity
☆ Vitamin deficiency
☆ Trace elements
☆ Age
☆ Obesity

6

Mangement of Tumours

S.K. Maiti

A tumour/neoplasm is caused by a purposeless multiplication of living cells. The word neoplasm means new growth. Tumours are common in carnivores as compared to other animals. Horse and cattle are mostly affected than sheep, pigs and goats. Old animals are affected more commonly than young ones. Cancer, according to current opinion, is a multitude of different diseases and is no more a "one disease'. Myriads of tumour types and plethora of their patho-physiology in different species necessitates species wise study of tumours in detail.

The etiology of tumours is not well established. Certain types of tumours are caused by viruses, chemicals, hormonal imbalances and gene mutations etc.

Clinically tumours may be classified into two types, benign or simple tumours and malignant tumours. A benign tumour does not recur after removal, whereas a malignant tumour does recur.

Type of Tumours

Connective Tissue Tumours

☆ *Fibroma*: consists of white connective tissue fibres, usually well capsulated and easy to remove

☆ *Chondroma*: composed of cartilaginous tissue

☆ *Osteoma*: composed of bony tissue

☆ *Odontoma*: composed of tooth tissue

☆ *Epulis*: arise from bone and periosteum at the alveolar border

☆ *Myoma*: made up of muscular tissue, *e.g.*, rhabdodomyoma-affecting the tongue

☆ *Myxoma*: structure resembles connective tissue and vitreous humour of the eye

☆ *Lipoma*: composed of fat cells

☆ *Neuroma*: made up of nerve cells and fibres

☆ *Glioma*: composed of neurogenic tissue

☆ *Angioma*: made up of lymphatic or blood vessels

☆ *Sarcoma*: malignant tumour involving any kind of connective tissue like bone, cartilage, fibrous tissue etc.

Epithelial Tumours

☆ *Papilloma*: tumour originating from the epithelium of the skin or mucous membranes appearing in the form of a wart-like growth from the surface.

☆ *Adenoma*: epithelial tumour with a gland like structure originating from glandular epithelium, eg. adenoma of salivary gland.

☆ *Carcinoma*: malignant epithelial tumour ; *e.g.*, carcinoma of eye, mammary gland etc.

Endothelial Tumours

☆ *Mesothelioma*: develops from mesothelial tissue

☆ *Perithelioma*: develops from the tunica adventitia of blood vessels

☆ *Psammoma*: fibrous tumour of brain tissue

☆ *Cholesteatoma*: tumour of crystalline structure; *e.g.*, cholesteatoma of brain.

Lymphoid Tissue Tumour

☆ *Lymphoma*: tumour made up of lymphoid tissue

☆ *Lymphosarcoma*: malignant neoplasm arising in lymphatic tissue

☆ *Teratoma:* a tumour containing disorderly arranged tissues and organs, resulting from faulty embryonic differentiation and organisation

☆ *Dermoid cyst*: a tumour composed of cutaneous tissues

☆ *Dentigerous cyst*: a tumour containing tooth

Diagnosis

☆ By their gross appearance

☆ *Benign tumour:* slow in growth, not adherent to overlying skin, usually do not ulcerate, not invade or infiltrate into surrounding tissue

☆ *Malignant tumour:* grows rapidly and gives rise to secondary tumours in their vicinity and in other parts of the body, skin is usually adherent to the tumour and may ulcerate

☆ *Histopathological examination*: malignant tumour- the cells constituting the tumour are immature and are in a state of active multiplication.

Prognosis

A benign tumour is not harmful except when it is large enough to cause mechanical pressure on the surrounding tissues/organs and interfere with their functions. They may be successfully excised/removed. Malignant tumours in the great majority of cases are incurable.

Treatment

- ✩ *Ligation*: a tight ligature is applied at the base of the tumour so as to cut the blood supply. The tumour sloughs off within 10-15 days. Ligation is convenient only in the case of pedunculated tumours.

- ✩ *By using red-hot iron*: the tumour is clamped below its base and the red-hot iron is applied distal to the clamp so as to remove the tumour. By this method, removal is possible without much haemorrhage.

- ✩ *By using ecraseur*: the ecraseur is useful specially for removing small pedunculated tumours situated in the pharynx, vagina etc. The tumour is held within the chain loop and is tightened around the base of the tumour to effect removal.

- ✩ *Chemical caustics*: chemicals like caustic potash, arsenical paste, nitric acid, acetic acid etc. may be used for removal of small tumours. Salicylic acid ointment is very effective for warts.

- ✩ *Surgical excision*: the tumour is carefully dissected out from the surrounding tissues under local or regional anaesthesia. Care should be taken to remove all the tumour cells, at the same time there should not be too much damage to the surrounding tissues. If the surrounding lymph glands are involved, they should also be removed.

- ✩ *Treatment for warts*: larger warts may be enucleated surgically. The use of "wart vaccine" is found useful in certain cases in bovines. A 20-25 ml of the vaccine is given subcutaneously and is repeated once or twice at weekly intervals (vaccine preparation protocol: remove few warts, triturate them in normal saline, leave at room temperature, remove supernatant fluid, heat to 50°C for one hr-add 5-10 per cent phenol-formalin. The dose is 5-10 ml s.c.) Medical grade DMSO has also been successfully used for removal of warts. Single application usually assures gradual disappearance of warts.

- ✩ *Treatment for malignant tumours*: treatment is useless in the case of malignant tumours because of their tendency to recur. But temporary relief may be afforded by total excision of the tumour. Amputation of the affected part is sometime advisable when the tumour is situated on extremities like limbs, tail and penis. Combination of surgery along with chemotherapy/radiotherapy also can be practised.

- ✩ *Cryotherapy*: cryogenic technique is used to freeze and cause necrosis and sloughing of tumour tissues. A cryoprobe, which is in the form of a hollow metal rod, is used for this purpose. Liquid or gaseous nitrous oxide

(−70°C) or liquid nitrogen (-180°C) is circulated. To destroy tumours of the skin, mouth and pharynx, it can be utilized.

Canine Mammary Tumour (CMT)

Of all species, dog develops neoplasm twice as frequently as humans, with incidence of skin and mammary tumours being the highest. Tumours of mammary gland are the most common tumours of female dog representing about 30-50 per cent of all tumours and it is the second most common tumour after skin neoplasm and most common malignant tumour in dogs.

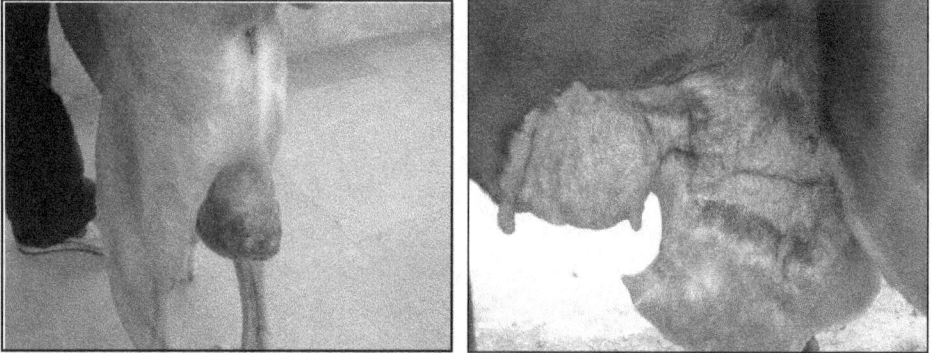

Figure 6.1: Venereal Tumour and Mammary Tumour in Dogs

Dogs have 5 mammary glands on each side (total of 10 breasts)-cranial thoracic, caudal thoracic, cranial abdominal, caudal abdominal and inguinal. The normal gland should be soft and pliant, especially towards the rear legs. There should be no firm lumps. Posterior mammary glands (4th and 5th) are often involved (about 65 per cent) compared to their anterior counter parts. The reason for this is that the posterior glands are having greater volume of breast tissue. Both benign and malignant tumours are more frequent in posterior glands with an incidence of 32.7 per cent and 35.6 per cent in caudal abdominal and inguinal mammary gland, respectively.

High risk breeds: Poodle, English Spaniel, English setter, Terriers and German shepherd.

Low- risk breeds: Boxer, Chihuahua, Greyhounds and Beagles.

Mammary tumours occur almost exclusively in female dogs. However, there are several reports of its occurrence in male dogs, which are usually very aggressive and have a poor prognosis.

The incidence increases with age of animals. The median age at diagnosis is between 10 and 12 years. Occasionally, it may be found in animals as young as 2 years. These tumours are rare in dogs that were spayed at less than 2 years of age.

The etiology of spontaneous mammary neoplasia in dog is unknown. But several studies have been conducted to unveil this enigma. The risk reducing effect of early ovariohysterectomy, in development of mammary tumour in dog is well documented. Development of mammary neoplasm is hormone dependent, with risk in bitches spayed before first estrus, after one estrus and after 2 or more cycles being 0.5 per cent, 8 per cent and 26 per cent, respectively. A higher risk for mammary cancer has been reported for multifarious bitches and in animals that have had few litters compared to those which have whelped large number of litters. Incriminating factors put forth for etiological significance of mammary tumour in dogs are sex hormonal derangement, higher growth hormone level, use of progestins for estrus control and β-type retroviral particles and BRCA-1/2 gene mutations.

Mammary tumours present as a solid mass or as multiple swelling. When tumours first appear they look like small pieces of pea gravel just under the skin. They are very hard and difficult to move around under the skin. They can grow rapidly in a short period of time, doubling their size every month or so. When tumours do arise in the mammary tissue, they are usually easy to detect by gently palpating the mammary glands. It usually occurs most frequently in the 4th and 5th mammary gland. In half of the cases, more than one growth is observed. Multiple glands in one or both mammary chains may be affected. Cystic ducts associated with the tumour may cause fluid secretion through the nipple. Lymphatic involvement may cause local swelling (lymph oedema) and discomfort, especially in the hind legs. Respiratory or other organ metastases may result in systemic problems (*e.g.*, dyspnea, anorexia, vomiting and diarrhoea). Benign growths are often smooth, small and slow growing. Signs of malignant tumours include rapid growth, irregular shape, firm attachment to the skin or underlying tissue, bleeding and ulceration. Occasionally tumours that have been small for a long period of time may suddenly grow quickly and aggressively, but this is an exception and not the rule.

It is very difficult to determine the type of tumour based on physical inspection. A biopsy or tumour removed is always needed to determine if the tumour is benign or malignant, and to identify what type it is. Tumours, which are more aggressive may metastasize and spread to the surrounding lymph nodes or to the lungs. A chest X-ray and physical examination of the lymph nodes will often help in confirming malignancy.

Diagnosis

- ☆ *History:* rate of growth, reproductive history, medication history and other systemic disorders
- ☆ Documentation and measurement of all mammary gland lesions
- ☆ Pre-surgical haematological and biochemical profile, as for the geriatric patient
- ☆ Thoracic radiography, including two lateral and one dorso-ventral view for metastasis
- ☆ *Cytology:* abnormal teat secretions-rarely diagnostic for neoplasia may be septic mastitis, fine needle aspiration from lesions-positive for carcinoma-

consider more radical initial surgery; negative-does not rule out malignancy

☆ *Biopsy*: eliminates all gross evidence of disease.

☆ Histopathology of tumours: benign, malignant or mixed.

Clinical Staging of Canine Mammary Carcinoma (WHO Classification)

T   T1-Less than 3 cm diameter

T2-3-5 cm diameter

T3-Greater than 5 cm in diameter

Subgroups

a) Not fixed to other tissues

b) Fixed to skin

c) Fixed to underlying muscle

T4- Any size, but inflammatory carcinoma (dermal infiltration)

N   N0-No nodal involvement

N1a- Ipsilateral node, nonfixed

N1b- Ipsilateral node-fixed

N2a- Bilateral nodes, nonfixed

N2b-Bilateral node-fixed

M   M0- No distant metastasis

M1- Metastatic

Stage-I: T0, T1 a, b, or c, N0, M0

Stage-II: T0, T1 or T2, a b. or c, N0 or N1a, M0

Stage-III: Any T3 tumour, with any N, and M0; Status or any T with Nb and M0

Stage-IV: Any T, Any N and M1 status

where, T= Tumor; N= Node; M= Metastasis

Treatment

Surgery

Surgery stands as first choice for the treatment of canine mammary tumours. The simplest surgical procedure in the mammary gland should be performed in the absence of metastatic disease and inflammatory carcinoma. Six categories of surgical excision of mammary tumours had been reported.

☆ Removal of tumour alone (lumpectomy)

☆ Removal of gland bearing tumour (simple mastectomy)

☆ Removal of tumour, gland intervening lymphatic and regional lymph node (en-bloc dissection)

☆ Removal of gland and adjacent gland 1 of 2 or 4 of 5 (half chain removal)

☆ Removal of entire chain of 5 mammary glands + regional lymph node (unilateral mastectomy)

☆ Removal of all 10 mammary glands, the skin covering them and the four lymph nodes at the same time (radical mastectomy).

The goal of surgery in canine mammary cancer is to remove all tumours by simplest procedure. More surgery is not better surgery for the dog. Upon finding any mass within the breast of a dog, surgical removal is recommended unless the patient is very old.

☆ If a single gland is affected, then only that gland is removed

☆ If multiple glands on one side are affected, then the entire 5 glands on that side are removed

☆ If multiple glands have tumours on both sides then both mammary chains are removed (all 10 glands are removed)

☆ If the lymph nodes (axillary/inguinal) are within the resection zone, then they also are removed and especially if they are enlarged

☆ If a growth is detected in the number 2 gland on the left side, glands 1, 2, and 3 and the axillary lymph node on that side should be removed

☆ If it is found in the number 4 gland on the right side, then glands 3, 4, 5, and the inguinal lymph node on that side should be completely removed

☆ If the groin region is difficult to suture closed, a flap of skin from the flank may be needed to reconstruct the area

Chemotherapy

If the tumour is malignant or shows evidence of invasion into the lymphatic system or blood vessels, chemotherapy should be recommended. The recommended dosage of different chemotherapeutic agents is as follows:

☆ *Cyclophosphamide* 0.3 mg/kg, IV for 14 days and then rest for 14 days

☆ *Chlorambucil* 0.2 to 0.3 mg orally daily for 2 months

☆ 5- *Fluorouracil* 5 mg/kg IV for 5 days then weekly

☆ *Vincristine* 0.1 to 0.5 mg/kg IV daily

☆ *Doxorubicin* 30 mg/sq. m IV 21 days apart up to 4-8 treatments

☆ *Tamoxifen* 20-40 mg/day orally in two divided doses for 1-3 weeks

☆ *Methotrexate* 0.65 mg/kg IV at weekly intervals for 2-4 weeks

☆ *Nanosomal Paclitaxel* 150 mg/32 kg b.wt on days 0/21/42

☆ *Nanosomal Docetaxel* 30 mg/32 kg b.wt on days 0/21/42

Prognostic Factors

☆ If a dog is spayed before the first estrous cycle there is about 0-0.5 per cent chance that this dog will develop mammary cancer

☆ Spaying a dog after the 4th estrous cycle or after 2.5 yr of age will not decrease the risk for developing mammary cancer

☆ After a dog has mammary cancer, spaying the animal does not decrease the recurrence rate of the cancer, as these tumours are not under the influence of estrogen

☆ The larger the mammary tumour the greater is the risk that it has spread to the lymph nodes, lungs or other parts of the body

☆ When a mammary tumour is found, there is 50 per cent chance that it is malignant and 50 per cent chance that it is benign

☆ Of the malignant mammary tumours, 50 per cent have already spread at the time of diagnosis

☆ If a dog has multiple tumours, some may be malignant and some may be benign

☆ If the tumour is less than 3 cm in size the recurrence rate is relatively low, and if greater than 3 cm the recurrence rate is fairly high

☆ If the biopsy indicates that the mammary tumour has spread to the lymph nodes, lymphatic channels or blood vessels, the prognosis is poor

☆ If the biopsy indicates that the tumour is surrounded by lymphocytes, a better prognosis is expected.

Complications

☆ Anesthetic death-rare

☆ Infection-rare

☆ Breakdown of the incision, which may require re-suturing of the wound or leaving it to heal on its own

☆ Spread of cancer to other regions of the body (lymph nodes, lungs, bones)

☆ Recurrence.

7

Affections of Horns

Aswathy Gopinathan and Kiranjeet Singh

The shape, built and contour of horn is a major criteria to characterize different breeds of indigenous Zebu cattle of India. The males with hefty horns are venerated for all ceremonies related to religion or agriculture. In sharp contrast to this, the cattle in countries with well developed bovine industry or organized dairy sector are routinely dehorned. Dehorning is one of the oldest and most common surgical procedures done in cattle. Dehorned cattle are safer for handlers and to other cattle. Apart from cattle welfare, this procedure is economically significant by preventing losses due to damage to the hide, safer while transport as well as marketing the livestock. Dehorning is an elective procedure except in cattle with fractured horns or osteomyelitis. Cosmetic dehorning is performed in somewhat mature animals which have a defective horn, or to treat accidental horn fractures or horn cancer.

Anatomy

The modified epithelium destined to become the future horn grows from the skin as "horn buds". This can be very well felt as soft buttons on either side of the poll. Under this, the cornual process of the frontal bone grows and it takes nearly 2 months for the horn bud epithelium to attach to the developing cornual process on the frontal bone. The cornual process gets covered with the blood bearing corium and the cornified epithelium. At the time of dehorning a skin tissue of 1-1.5 cm around the base of horn also needs to be removed since there lies the germinal epithelium to horn. If this area is also removed, the haired skin will replace the defect without re-growth of horn.

Blood supply to the horn: Cornual artery, which is a branch of superficial temporal artery. Nerve supply to horn-cornual nerve a branch of zygomatic temporal nerve, which is a branch of the trigeminal nerve.

Restraint

Young animals can be straddled and held tight while the adult animals have to be restrained in a stanchion or in a chute with a head gate, the head tightly haltered and secured to minimize movement.

Anaesthesia

Two per cent lidocaine, loaded in a syringe with 18 gauge, 1-1.5 inch needle, 3-10 ml/side is injected half way between the lateral canthus of the orbit and base of the horn just under the shaft of frontal crest to block the cornual nerve and wait for 5-10 minutes. Aberrant innervations can often lead to lack of proper anaesthesia. Alternately, 100 mg xylazine added to 100 ml lidocaine administered locally at the rate of 0.1 mg/kg, half the dose at the base of each horn will provide adequate sedation in fractious animals.

Technique for Dehorning

It can be chemical, thermal or cutting.

Chemical Dehorning

A paste of sodium hydroxide, potassium hydroxide or calcium hydroxide applied at the area of buds, monitoring the animal so that the paste do not gravitate towards the eyes.

Thermal Dehorning

It is useful in small calves, where the dehorner can be entirely fit into the base of the horn bud. Portable electric dehorners are used on a shaven bud to make a circular cut around with adequate pressure and a twist upwards scoops the horn bud out. It must be done long enough to see a complete white rim of bone under the base of the burned bud to ensure that the blood supply to the horn bud is completely cut off.

In young animals that have missed the early disbudding procedure, it can be achieved through different devices like cutting dehorner (saw/obstetrical wire) or gouging forceps.

Cosmetic Dehorning (Amputation of Horn)

It allows primary closure of the skin after removing the horn for achieving a cosmetic appearance. It produces less scarring than the above mentioned techniques, requires less healing time and can be performed in mature animals. Anaesthesia is achieved by infiltrating 5-10 ml of 5 per cent lidocaine in fan shape, under the frontal ridge half way between the lateral canthus of the eye and base of horn. All the animals require a hemi-circumferential infiltration of local anaesthetic on the caudal aspect of the horn base to anaesthetize cutaneous branches of second cervical spinal nerve. In adult goats both corneal and infratrochlear nerves supply to the horn. Cornual branch is blocked with 2-3 ml lidocaine half way between the lateral canthus of eye and the lateral horn base, as close as possible to the ridge of supraorbital process. Infratrochlear branch is desensitized by 2-3 ml lidocaine infiltrated half way between the medial canthus of eye and medial horn base, dorsal and parallel to the dorso-median aspect of the orbit. Infiltration should be done as a line block (maximum dose is 10 mg/kg in goats since they are sesnsitive to lidocaine toxicity). Administration of xylazine 0.05 mg/kg IV helps to sedate the animal.

Clip the hair around a wider area of horn base and pole. Elliptical incision is made leaving more than 1 cm margin around the base of horn, leaving 5-7 cm dorsal to and 5-7 cm ventral to the base of horn. The skin is dissected sharply from the underlying tissue in the ventral incision. An obstetrical wire is placed against the frontal bone at the ventral incision and directed towards the pole, and saw off the horn as close to the base of the horn as possible. Proper seating of the wire at the base of the horn is required to saw off the germinal epithelium at the horn base. Lavage the area with saline. The exposed cornual artery is ligated for haemostasis.The bone chips are removed and the area is washed thoroughly with normal saline. Undermine the skin to appose the wound edges. The skin edges are sutured by a series of simple interrupted sutures or mattress sutures with silk or nylon, and the sutures are kept for 2 -3 weeks.

Complications

Continuous bleeding cautions one to reopen the skin, pull the bleeder out and ligate it. A cotton pad soaked with tincture benzoin can be placed over the wound and kept until it is shed by its own. Any medication going into the sinus can cause severe irritation. Infection to the sinus can be prevented by undertaking proper aseptic technique. Sinusitis is a potential complication of this procedure; animals are produced with malodorous discharge from the site of dehorning, pyretic, anorexic and lethargic. The sinus should be opened and lavaged thoroughly with anti-inflammatory and antibiotic therapy for 2-3 weeks.

Chronic sinusitis can lead to bone osteomyelitis and sequestrum formation. Another unusual complication is skull fracture, when the instruments (saw) is not sharp and if undue pressure is exerted.

Horn Avulsion

This can occur due to trauma when the corium surrounding the horn core gets avulsed. The horn core is either intact or sometimes fractured, the main challenge is to control haemorrhage. A gauze bandage soaked with tincture benzion can be applied and let it remain there till shed off by its own. Fly repellants and anti-inflammatory drugs should be given for 1-2 weeks. If the horn is fractured, it can be amputed by any of the above said methods.

Horn Cancer

The squamous epithelial cells lining the base of the horn core can get converted to squamous cell carcinoma, this condition is usually seen in adult cattle 5-10 years old. The reasons can be multifactorial like trauma, radiation, chronic irritation etc. Higher prevalence of this condition is seen in castrated bullocks. Clinical signs are continuous shaking of the head, rubbing of horn against hard objects, slimy or bloody discharge from the nostrils or base of the horn, soft tumour mass exposing the horn from its base. Surgical removal of the horn can be attempted. Immunotherapy with tumour cells suspended in Freund's complete adjuvant can be injected subcutaneously at an interval of 5 days. Intra lesional injections of BCG or BCG cell wall extracts has also been tried with varying success rate.

8

Aural Haematoma in Dogs

J. Mohindroo

Aural haematoma or ear haematoma is one of the most common conditions encountered in small animal practice. It is the accumulation of blood, either fresh or clotted, within the pinna (ear flap). The ear flap is composed of a layer of skin on each side of a layer of cartilage. The cartilage gives the ear flap its shape. Blood vessels go from one side to the other by passing through the cartilage. The haematoma usually arises as a self-inflicted injury from scratching and head shaking. Violent shaking causes the vessels to rupture and bleed into the space between the ear cartilage and skin. Other reasons for the dogs shaking their ears may include bite wounds and otitis externa. Dogs with long, pendulous ears are at greater risk for developing ear haematoma. Dogs with clotting or bleeding disorders may also develop haematomas, with or without a history of trauma. When a haematoma is present, the pinna will appear very thick and spongy (Figure 8.1).

The swelling may involve the entire pinna or it may involve only one area. The swelling may occasionally become large and painful, and at times may occlude the opening of the ear canal. The extra weight of the ear flap may be uncomfortable and may lead to a permanent change in the cartilage of the ears and the affected ear may drop down permanently. Diagnosis usually can be made on palpation and physical examination. Whenever a dog is presented with ear haematoma it is important to address the underlying cause before initiating the treatment.

Surgical drainage is considered the most acceptable method of treating aural haematoma in dogs. The surgery is done under general anaesthesia, which may be induced with protocols which are well described in the standard books. It is preferred to pre-anaesthetise the animal with a combination of Butorphanol 0.2

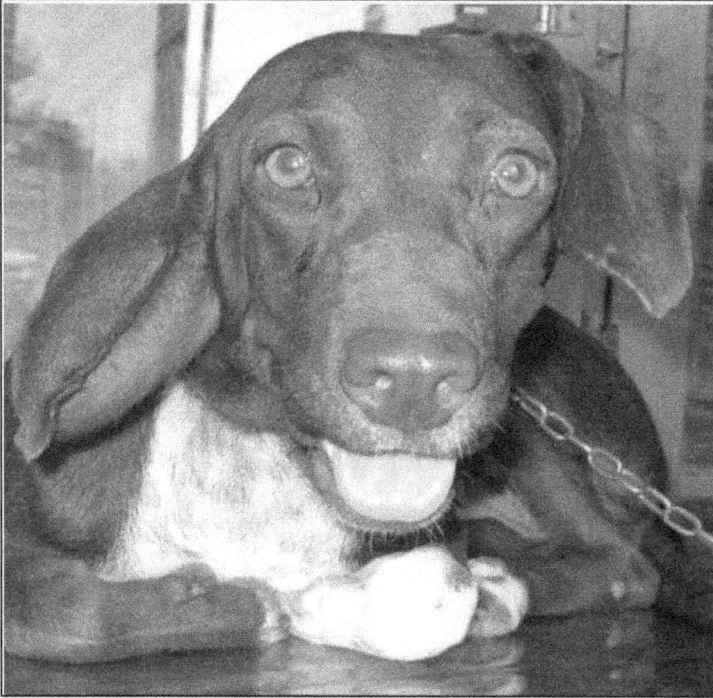

Figure 8.1: Haematoma of the Right Ear Showing Swelling of the Ear.

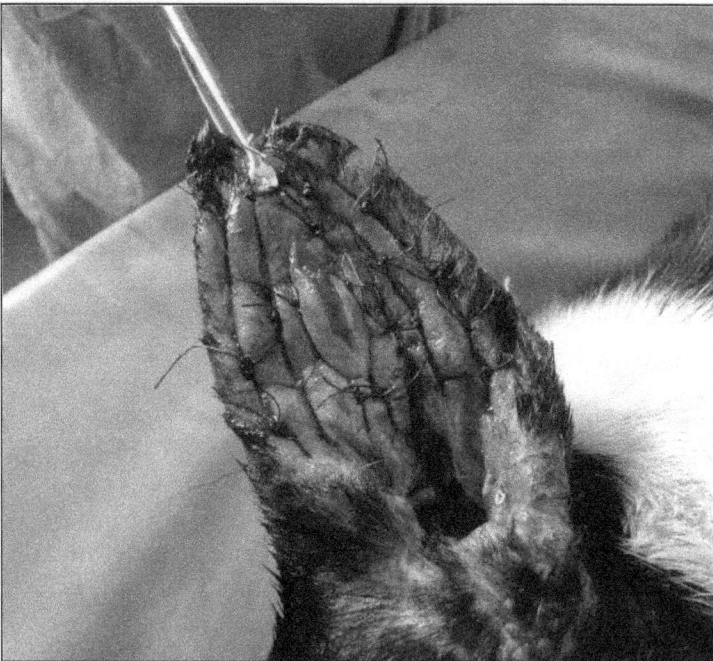

Figure 8.2: Application of Multiple Horizontal Mattress Sutures Using Nylon.

mg/kg b.wt, Acepromazine 0.05 mg/kg b.wt and Glycopyrrolate 0.01 mg/kg b.wt mixed in a single syringe and administered intramuscularly. Anaesthesia is then induced using 5 per cent Thiopental sodium 8-10 mg/kg b.wt i/v and maintained with 1-2 per cent Isoflurane using Boyle's apparatus (inhalation anaesthesia machine with partial re-breathing system. Under the field condition the dog may be anaesthetised with a combination of Xylazine 1 mg/kg, Ketamine 5 mg/kg and Atropine sulphate 0.045 mg/kg administered intramuscularly. Endotracheal intubation should be done prior to the start of surgery to provide a patent airway. The affected ear is kept uppermost and the ear is shaved and prepared for aseptic surgery. The ear canal is plugged with sterile gauze prior to making incision. A linear incision is then made on the concave surface of the ear pinna to drain the haematoma completely. An 'S' shaped or a diamond shaped incision may also be made to facilitate drainage of the haematoma. After completely evacuating the haematoma, the fibrin and clots are removed, and the cavity is freshened with a sterile gauze piece. The cavity should then be flushed with povidone iodine (betadine) before closure. Closure of the cavity is accomplished by placing multiple through and through sutures using a non absorbable suture material (nylon) in a horizontal mattress fashion (staple sutures) starting from the periphery to the incision line (Figure 8.2). After applying a series of sutures, care is taken to keep the

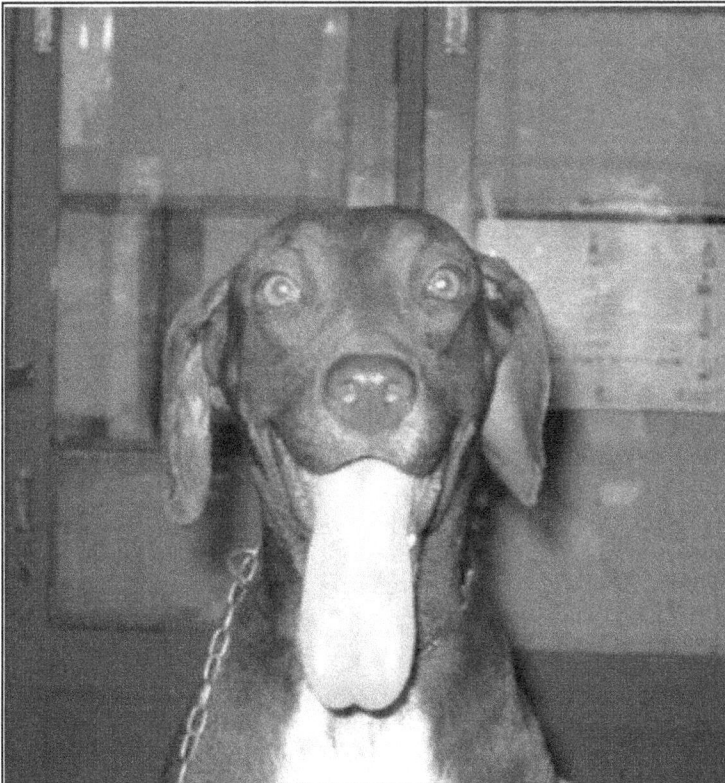

Figure 8.3: Good Cosmetic Outcome after Surgical Treatment of Haematoma.

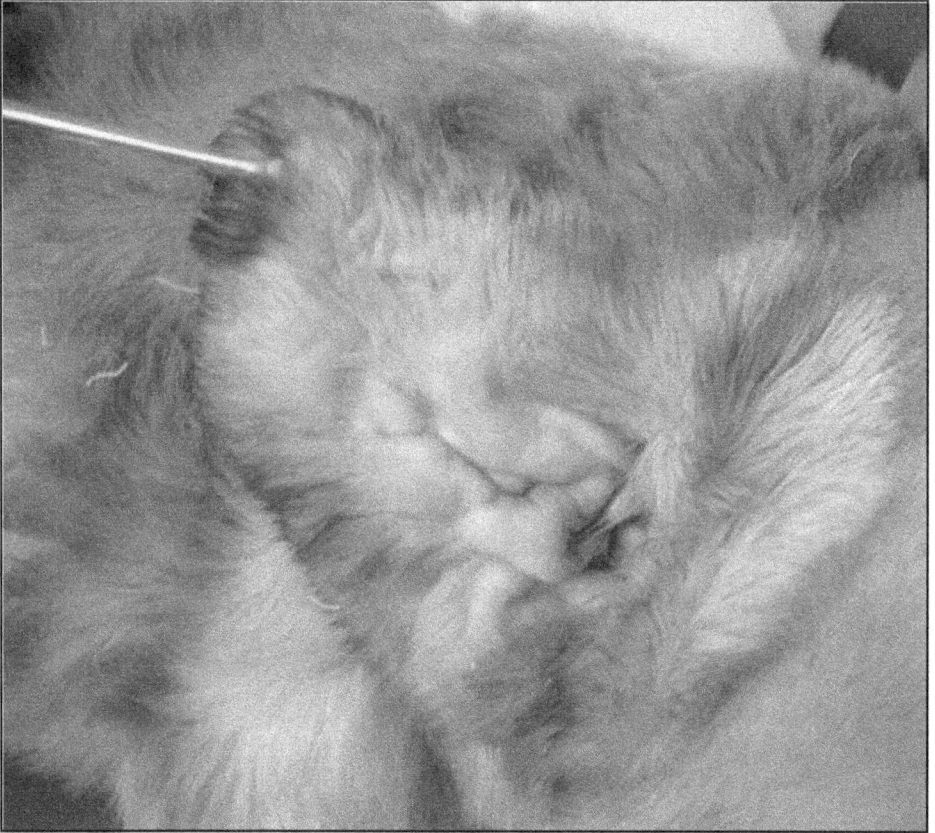

Figure 8.4: Wrinkling of the Ear after Surgical Treatment of Haematoma.

incision line gaping so as to facilitate continuous drainage of any fluids that may tend to accumulate. The ear pinna is then bandaged after placing rolls of cotton bandage/card board/X-ray film or any other stiff material on both sides, and then pressing the ear pinna against the dorsum of the head. This would provide sufficient pressure to prevent recurrence of the haematoma and maintain the integrity and shape of the ear pinna. Good bandaging technique usually prevents the complications of wrinkling/puckering and dropping of the ear pinna. The sutures are removed after 3 weeks. The cosmetic outcome with this method is usually good (Figure 8.3). Despite being recognised as one of the best methods of treatment of ear haematoma, surgical treatment may be associated with complications like wrinkling and puckering of the ear (Figure 8.4), drooping of the pinna and further damage to cartilage of pinna leading to permanent deformity.

Many other techniques (surgical and conservative) have been tried for treatment of ear haematoma *viz.* needle aspiration, administration of corticosteroids and gentamicin after aspiration, iodoform wick placement after incising the haematoma, malleable silicon lined ear dressings and placement of teat cannulas and catheters. Silicon, latex, PVC drains, carbon dioxide lasers and recently stainless

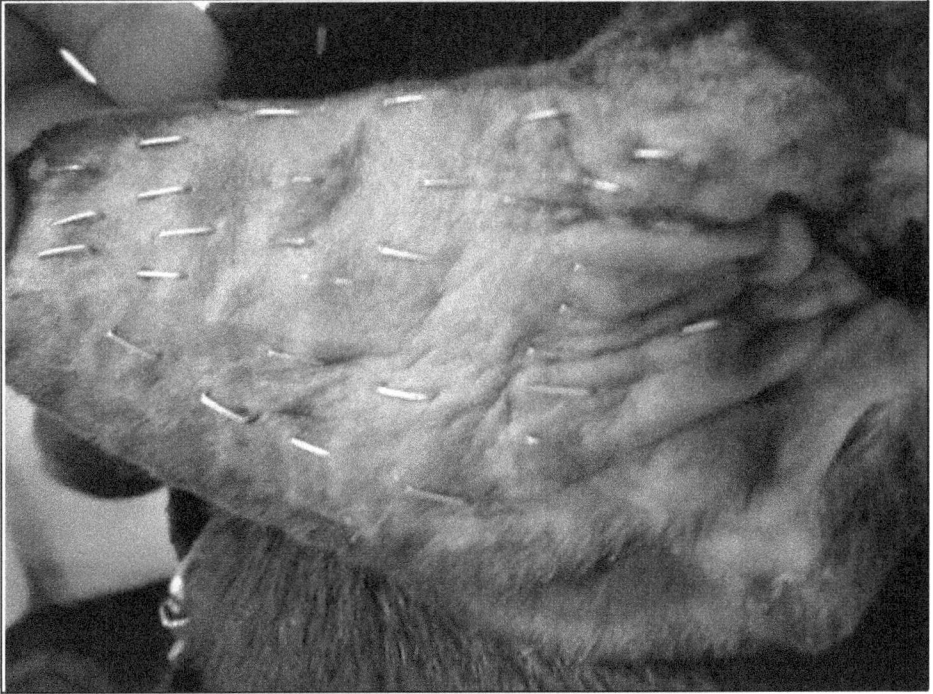

**Figure 8.5: Stainless Steel Skin Staples Applied on
Medial Surface of the Ear Pinna after Complete Healing.**

steel staples have also been used. However, all the techniques have certain limitations. Needle aspiration might lead to re-accumulation of blood/fluid, severe crumpling and scarring of the ear. Glucocorticoids further separate auricular cartilage and delay healing. Dressings also might not provide sufficient pressure and are considered inappropriate for large haematomas. Cannulas and catheters cause irritation and there is potential for continuous serosanguinous discharge from the tube. Drains like PVC and latex have been reported to cause drooping and disfiguration of ear pinna due to shrinking, fibrosis and cartilage erosion. Stainless steel skin staples applied on the concave aspect of the haematoma (Figure 8.5) have proved to be a fast technique, which requires less than a minute to complete the surgery. However, the cost of the staples is a limiting factor. Another limitation with the stainless steel staples is that it cannot be used in haematomas where the skin/cartilage is very thick.

Cyanoacrylates have also been tried, but intense granuloma formation discouraged their use.

9

Management of Basic Eye Affections in Animals

S.P. Tyagi

Though the management of various eye disorders in animals require a thorough specialized subject training of post-graduate level but in India due to the lack of the concepts of veterinary ophthalmic referral centres manned by Veterinary ophthalmologists, the field vets have to be adequately trained to deal with such cases at their own level or at least to manage initial treatment in a proper manner. This process requires not only acquiring the necessary surgical skills but also ensuring availability of commensurate basic diagnostic and therapeutic infrastructure. With such enabling support, most of the ocular problems of animals including intimidating emergencies can be successfully treated at field level with a surprising ease. The present report deals with some of such common eye problems of animals briefly:

Ocular Worms

Different kinds of slender worms can be observed in the eyes of different species of animals causing a variety of symptoms.

The most common worm infestation by '*Thelazia* spp.' is caused by 'face fly' feeding on ocular secretions. The dogs are commonly affected. The female worms residing in conjunctival sac of the infected animal discharge larvae in ocular secretions, which are ingested up by the face fly. Theses ingested larvae become third stage larvae within few weeks and appear in the salivary secretions of flies and deposited in host's eye during feeding and once inside conjuntival sac, they mature within few weeks.

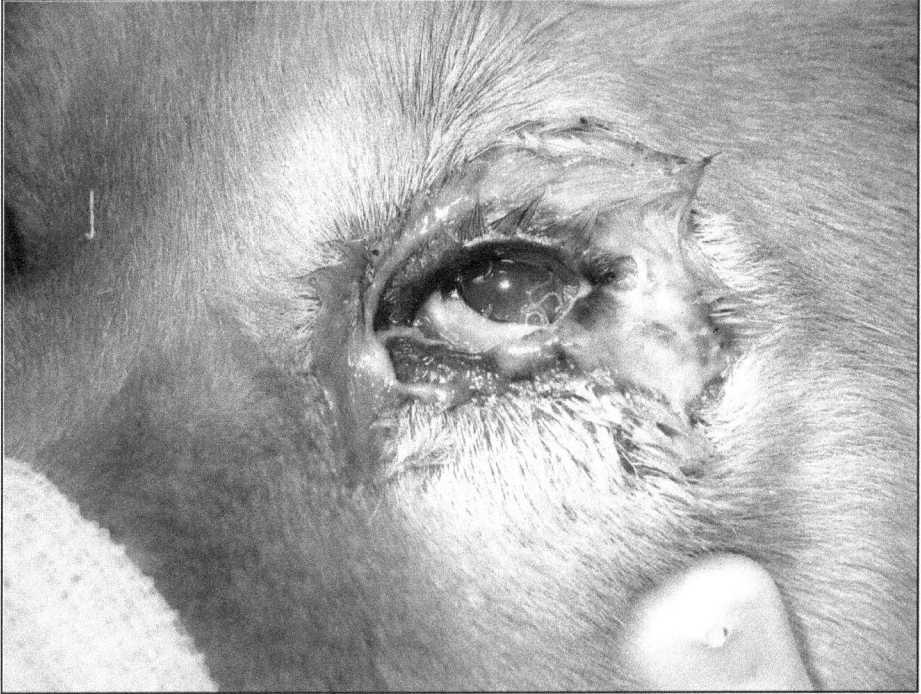

Figure 9.1: *Thelazia callipaeda* **within Conjunctival Sac of a Dog.**

Though majority of animals remain asymptomatic, but some show various clinical symptoms particularly when the worm load is heavy. The signs are: epiphora, conjunctivitis, frequent rubbing of eyes, corneal opacities, thick mucoid discharge and occasionally corneal ulcers. The infection may remain present all through the year.

Physical examination of the conjunctival sac after protracting the third eyelid usually immediately shows the presence of such worms in the affected animal. The worms are white or creamy coloured with a length ranging from few millimetres to about 2 cms. Occasionally some of the worms come out of conjunctival sac and may be observed slithering over the cornea and sclera. The worms are usually multiple. The worms may be removed manually by picking up with a serrated ophthalmic forceps and flushed with BSS. The secondary lesions of the eye generally heal spontaneously but may be appropriately treated, if needed. Systemic ivermectin, doramectin and levamisole are effective against such worms and can be used, though facial hygiene and strict fly control in endemic area are essential steps in proper prevention of this problem.

Occasionally another kind of eye-worm belonging to "*Setaria* spp." is also observed in different species of animals. The equines are commonly affected. Such worms are transmitted by the mosquito bites. These worms are predominantly found in the peritoneal cavity of the infected animal without causing much harm except occasional mild peritonitis. The larvae produced by these worms enter in to

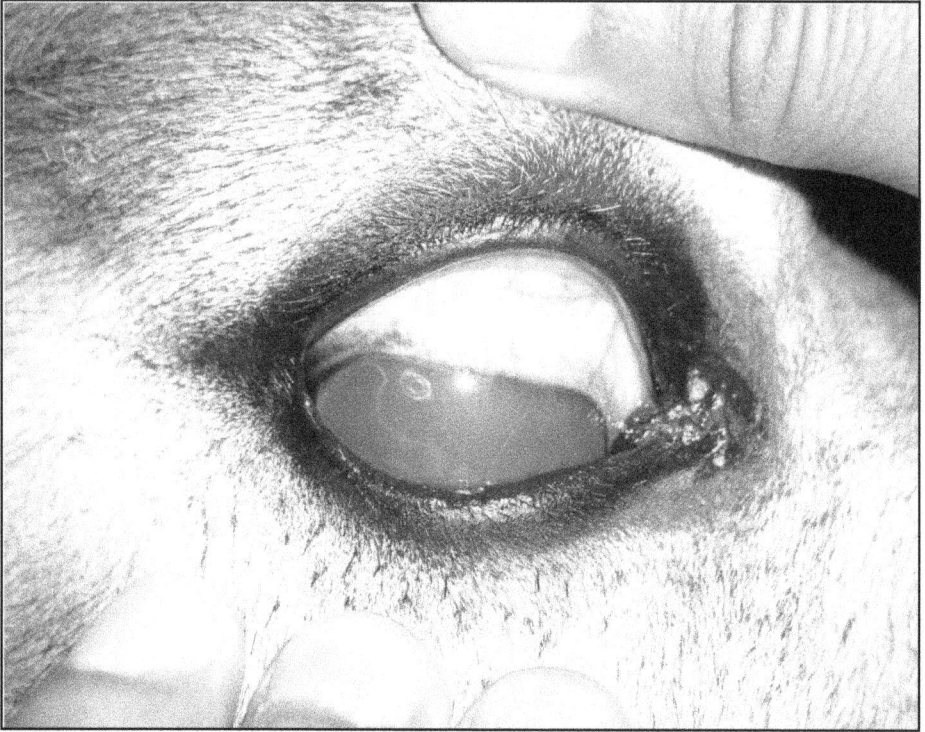

Figure 9.2: *Setaria equina* **inside Autinar Chamber of Eye in a Mule.**

the blood stream and ingested by mosquitoes during blood sucking. The larvae develop in the muscles of mosquitoes and become infective within 15 days and then appear in the saliva of mosquitoes. When such mosquitoes bite another animal, such infective larvae are transmitted. Occasionally young worm migrate to anterior chamber of the eye and cause severe inflammatory reactions.

The common clinical symptoms are epiphora and various degrees of corneal opacities. The other symptoms of uveitis will also be present. The naked eye examination generally easily reveals presence of slender thread-like whitish worm (mostly singule) wandering inside the anterior chamber of eye in the initial stages. However, spotting of worm is not easy when the corneal opacity worsens later on. The movement of worm may be stimulated by light, though it results in discomfort to the animal. In cases where worm is suspected but not visible due to complete corneal opacity, ophthalmic ultrasonography confirms the diagnosis.

The worm should be removed surgically before any anthelmintic is given because dead worm initiate sever immune mediated inflammatory response worsening corneal opacity. The procedure should be performed preferably under general anaesthesia (GA). The animal is secured in lateral recumbency after induction of GA. The eye is flushed with very dilute Povidone-iodine solution (5 per cent Betadine solution diluted with NS in a 1:50 ratio) and thoroughly lavaged with BSS after a few minutes. A few drops of 4 per cent Lignocaine are used to desensitize the cornea and a topical antibiotic-steroid combination (like Gatifloxacin-Prednisolone) is instilled over the eye. Suparorbital nerve block may be accomplished, if need be. The eyelid retractor is applied or alternatively eyeball is stabilized with three 4-0 sutures placed through Tenon's capsule approximately at 11, 3 and 7 O'clock position. A partial thickness clear corneal incision approximately 2 mm away from limbus is made in between 10 or 2 O'clock position of the cornea with a 2.8 mm ophthalmic crescent knife (though less preferred BP blade No. 11 can also be used for such incision). The anterior chamber is then entered with a stab force as soon as the worm comes near to the incision site and the knife is removed back with the same action. Simultaneously the eye ball is pressed from opposite side. The worm generally comes out easily along with the outflow of aqueous humour. In cases, where worm does not come out, the anterior chamber can be flushed with BSS like Ringer's lactate and the worm manually picked up using serrated ophthalmic forceps. If too much movement of worm causes problem in picking it up, sterile viscoelastic substance (*e.g.* Inj MIOSOL-PFS) can be injected into the anterior chamber to restrict its movement. Care must be taken not to force the worm deeper during this process, thus the canula of 'visco' injector should be under the worm and near the iris during injection. The stab incision up to 2.8 mm can be left as such without suturing. Post-operatively 2 drops each of topical antibiotic-steroid combination and a cycloplegic like 1 per cent Tropicamide may be instilled in the eye q.i.d. for a week. The topical ointments should be avoided for the first few days.

For destroying the circulating microfilariae and the adult worms at other places of body, suitable systemic anthelmintic should be used post-operatively.

Entropion

It is the inward rolling of the eyelid margin leading to corneo-scleral irritation because of rubbing of misdirected eyelid cilia. It may be developmental or cicatrical in origin or may be spastic occurring secondary to pain and blepherospasms. The dogs are commonly affected animal species.

The clinical symptoms are epiphora, rubbing of eye, mucopurulent discharge from the eye and photophobia. In chronic cases conjunctival congestion, corneo-scleral vascularization and corneal ulcers may develop. In cases of developmental entropion, the symptoms are not as distinct in initial stages as the cilia are softer.

Physical naked eye examination reveals the exact extent of entropion and either (commonly) a part of the eyelid margin or (less commonly) whole of the eyelid margin is found rolled inwards with its cilia touching the cornea. The lower eyelid is commonly affected.

The treatment consists of either eyelid tacking or surgical excision of lid tissue popularly known as 'Hotz Celsus' procedures.

The eyelid tacking is fit for neonates or very young patients up to 20 weeks of age. Maintaining eyelids in relatively normal position for a few weeks may sometimes resolve the problem permanently. Repeated tacking may be undertaken until maturity when if required, excisional procedure may be adopted. For simple

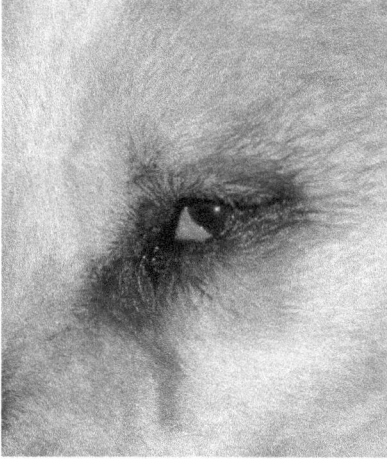

Figure 9.3: Entropion in a Dog towards Lateral Aspects of Lower Eyelid.

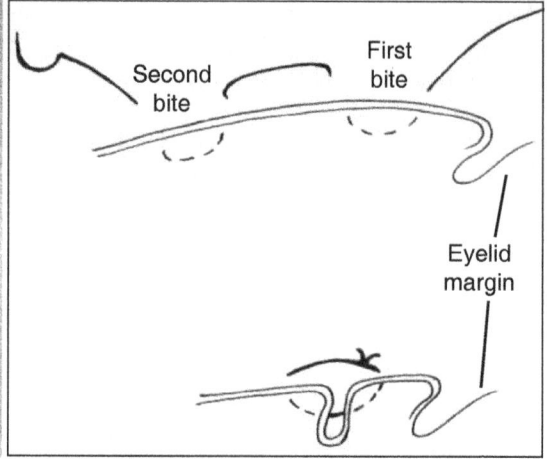

Figure 9.4: Eyelid Tacking using Inverted Lamber Suture.

eyelid tacking, the skin adjacent to entropion area is grasped with a tissue forceps and attached with adjacent skin using tissue adhesive, thus creating a little fold which evert the eyelid margin sufficient enough to correct the entropion.

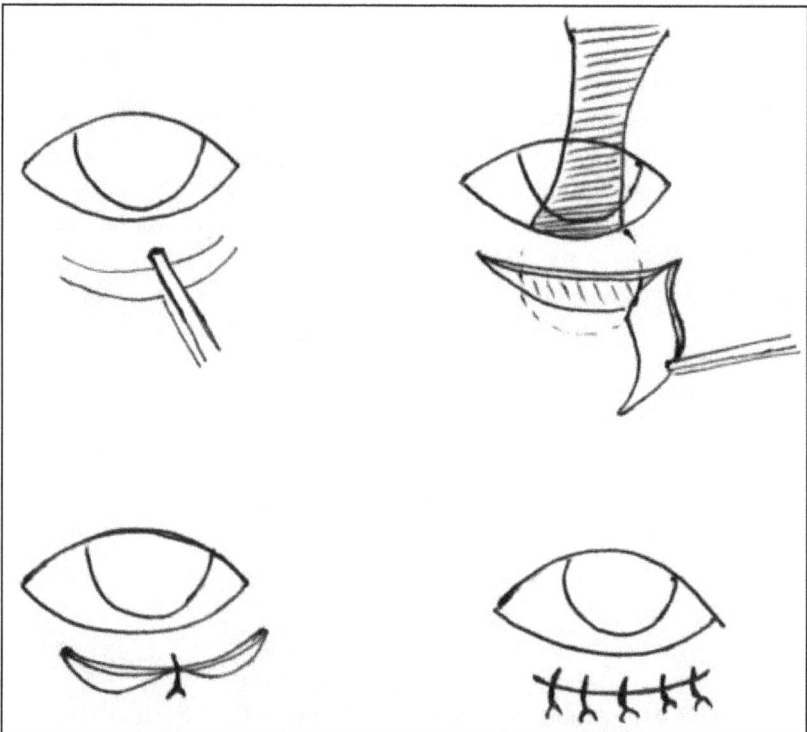

Figure 9.5: Techniques for Correction of Entropion in a Dog.

The eyelid tacking can also be done by applying inverted Lambert sutures at eyelid margins using non-absorbable 3-0 to 4-0 sutures with animal under GA. For this procedure, start suture bite from approximately 3 mm away from the eyelid margin, involve about 5 mm skin and orbicularis muscle in first bite; exit 5 mm away and take a second bite of about same 5 mm length involving skin and orbital fascia. Tie the suture and thus inverting a furrow of skin. A drop of tissue adhesive may be used additionally to stick the skin folds around the skin furrow.

In severe cases or in mature animals eyelid skin resection is necessary to correct entropion. The Hotz-Celsus or "pinch" procedure is most commonly used for this purpose.

With animal under GA the eyelid margin is grasped with a forceps to estimate the wedge area to be removed for correction of entropion. The eyelid is stabilized with an eyelid plate placed under conjunctival fornix, the eyelid is stretched and the wedge shaped area of skin estimated as explained above is excised using BP blade No. 15. The incision should be 1-3 mm away from the eyelid margin. The skin defect is closed by suturing the edges of skin with 4-0 non-absorbable interrupted sutures. Remember that 0.5-1.0 mm additional eversion of eyelid may occur during healing period; this fact should be taken into account while estimating the size and excising the skin wedge.

Elizabeth collar, topical antibiotic-steroid combination and systemic NSAID are to be used post-operatively for a few days.

Ectropion

It is the eversion of the lower eyelid margin commonly seen in dogs. It may be developmental or secondary to scar tissue formation or simply fatigue of orbicularis oculi muscle. In certain breeds like St. Bernard, the eyelids and palpebral fissure are excessive in size which predisposes the animal for ectropion.

The clinical symptoms arise because of exposure of bulbar and palpebral conjunctiva and inability of animal to channelize its tears in to nasolacrimal system efficiently. Thus epiphora, chronic keratitis, conjunctivitis or keratoconjunctivitis are observed in affected animal.

The common surgical treatment is 'V to Y eyelid plasty'. In this procedure, a V shaped piece of eyelid skin is removed just below the ectropion area. The base of this 'V' is kept towards eyelid margin starting about 1 mm below it. Now beginning at the most distal aspect of the 'V' incision the skin edges are closed together with simple interrupted 4-0 non-absorbable sutures; thus making the stem of the 'Y'. Working upwards the stem of 'Y' is lengthened until eyelid margin elevates to its normal position. Usually this length is 2-3 mm more than the actual ectropion area. Once the eyelids are in normal position, the remaining tissue defect is sutured to form arms of the 'Y'.

The post-operative care remains same as explained in entropion correction.

Remember, entropion and ectropion may occur simultaneously in the same animal in the same eye or in the same eyelid.

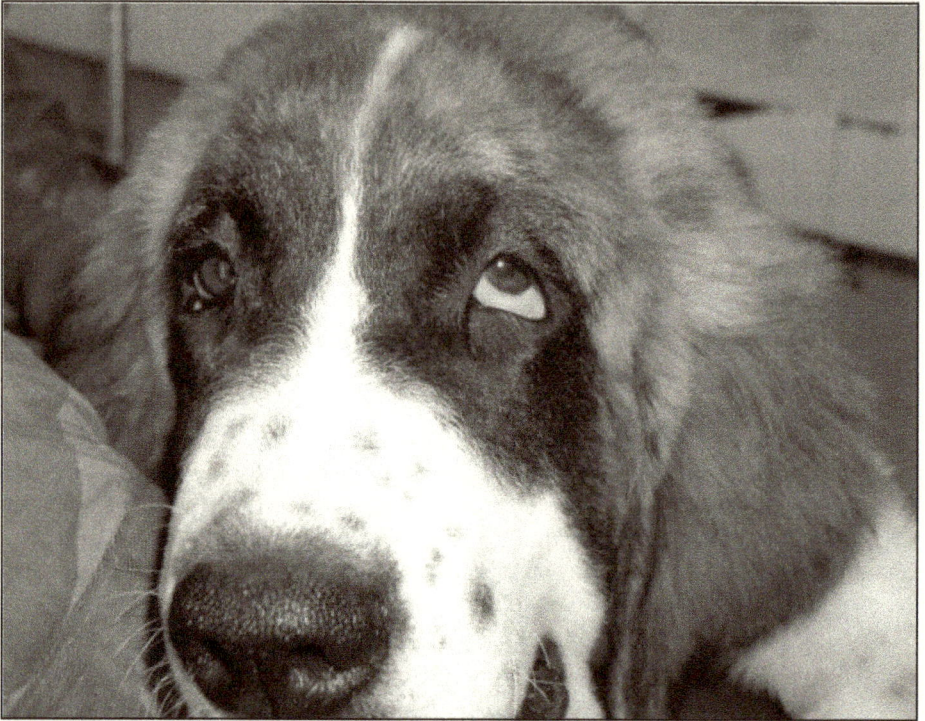

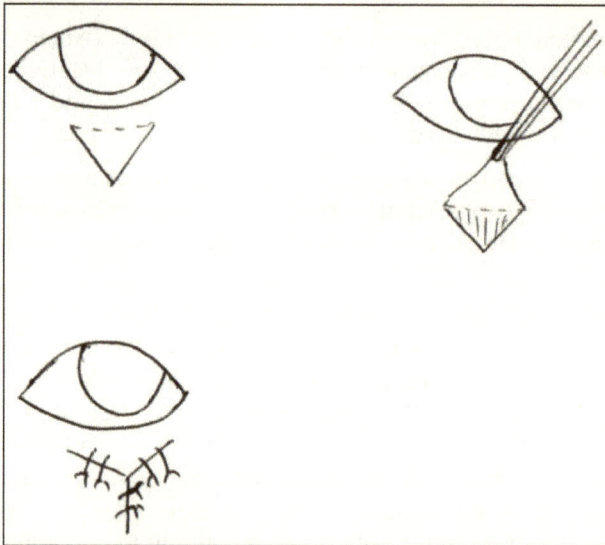

Figure 9.6: Ectropion in a Dog and V-Y Blepheroplasty for its Surgical Correction.

Cherry Eye

It is the protrusion of third eyelid gland in young dogs and cats. This results probably due to defect in the retinaculum, which anchors the gland in the periorbital region.

The clinical symptoms arise due to exposure of third eyelid and its subsequent desiccation causing irritation to the animal. Thus the symptoms are a visible fleshy mass towards medial canthus of eye accompanied with abnormal tear production and discharge; occasional rubbing of eye may lead to exposed tissue damage. The condition may be unilateral but most likely turns bilateral.

Medicinal treatment with topical antibiotic-steroid combination is helpful but seldom curative without surgical intervention. The preferred surgical option is one among many techniques to replace the gland in its normal position. The option of partial or complete excision of gland is reserved only for refractory cases because removal of third eyelid gland will deprive the animal of an important source of tears. This gland produces up to half of the total tear volume and thus animal will be predisposed to keratoconjunctivitis sicca (KCS) or 'dry eye' following this gland's excision. However, non-treatment of the condition for a long time will also incapacitate this gland to form tears and rather increase the chances of developing KCS compared to even early excisional options.

The common surgical options for gland replacement are conjunctival mucosa pocket technique, intra-nictitating tacking procedure and posterior (bulbar) nictitans anchoring techniques. Here the easier conjunctival mucosa pocket technique is described, which is suitable for small protruded masses.

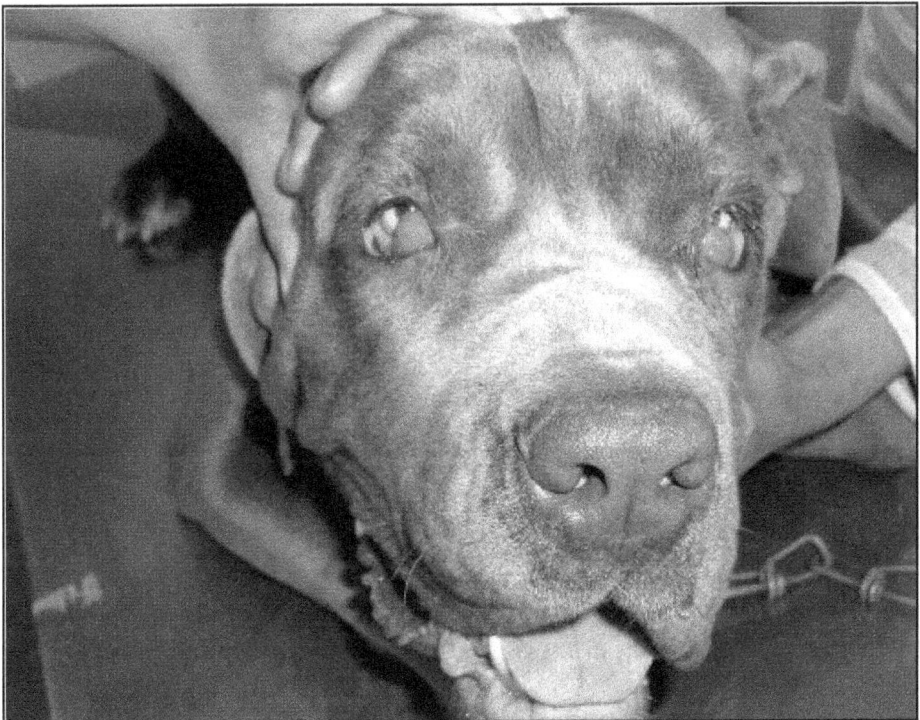

Figure 9.7: Cherry Eye in a Napolean Mastiff.

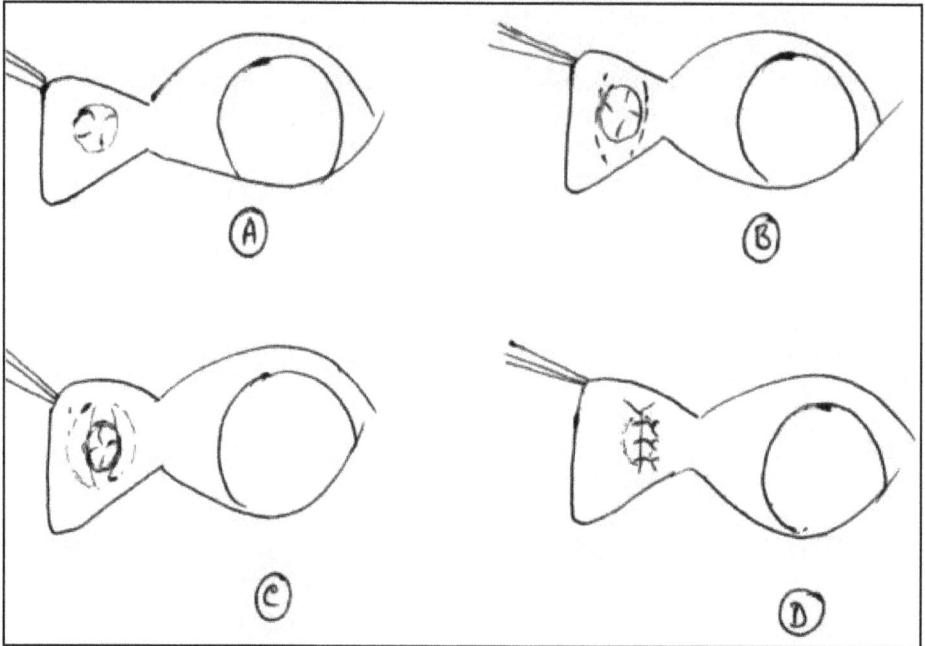

Figure 9.8: Conjunctival Mucosa Pocket Technique for Correction of Cherry Eye.

For this procedure, the animal is anaesthetized and secured in lateral recumbency with the affected side up; its third eyelid is grasped with thumb forceps and protracted forward to expose its bulbar surface. The third eyelid gland is identified and two curved incisions are given on conjunctiva mucosa on either side of this gland with the help of BP blade No. 15. The edges of these incisions are not joined. Now the central mucosal covering over gland is left undisturbed, whereas, little undermining of conjunctiva is done by directing the Steven's scissors away from gland to free up the incised conjunctival margins. These edges are now pulled over central gland and closed with 5-0 to 6-0 absorbable continuous sutures with buried knotting technique.

The post-operative care remains same as described above.

Remember cherry eye condition of Napolean Mastiff breed of dogs (Picture above) is not amenable to gland replacement procedures and thus need to be excised for treatment.

Dermoids

Ocular dermoids are characterized by island/s of skin that are histologically normal but are located at abnormal places like cornea, sclera, nictitating membrane, eyelids etc. Such affections are observed in all animal species sporadically.

The clinical symptoms are due to irritation of eye surface with the hairs of dermoid and thus include chronic epiphora, conjunctivitis and keratitis.

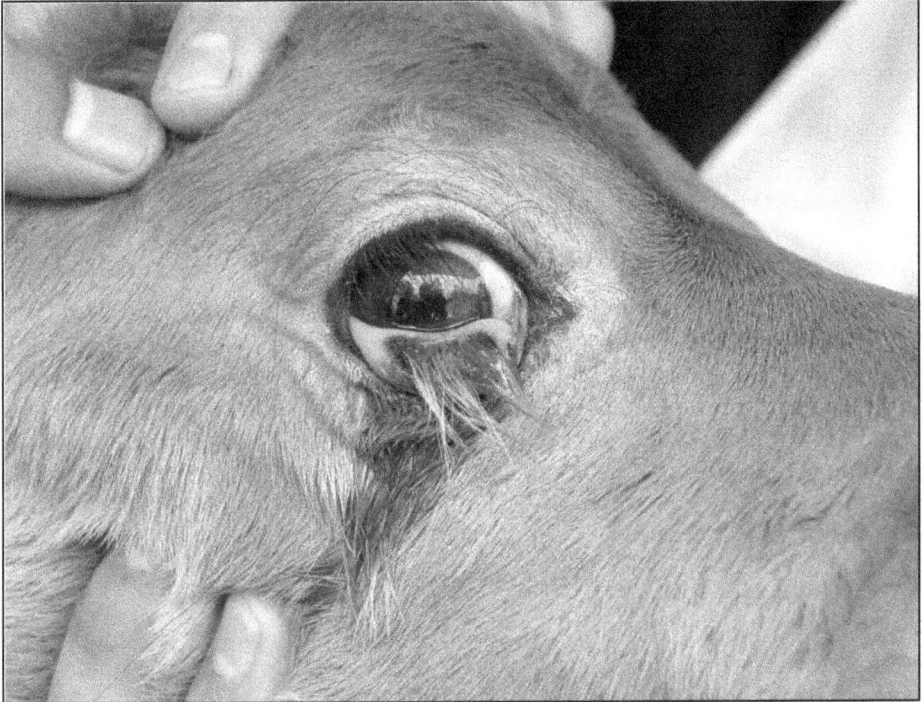

Figure 9.9: Dermoid involving Nictitating Membrane in a Calf.

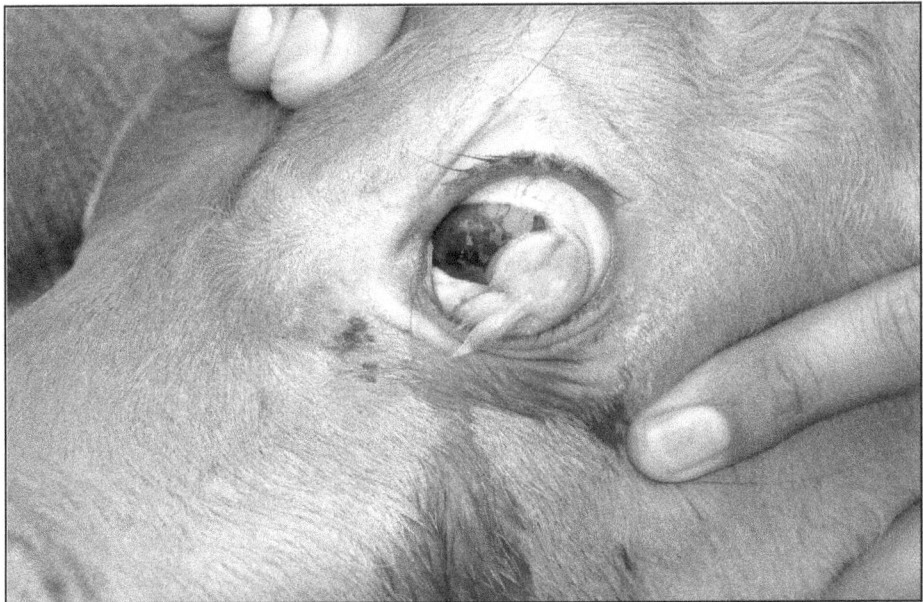

Figure 9.10: Dermoid Involving Cornea and Selena in a Calf.

The treatment is surgical excision of the complete growth. If the dermoid involves cornea, then the surgery is to be performed by an experienced ophthalmic surgeon as it may involve technically more demanding partial keratectomy.

Foreign Bodies in the Eye

Penetrating or non-penetrating, both kinds of foreign bodies (FB) may cause severe damage to the eye in animals. Some smaller foreign bodies may get lodged under the eyelids and continue to irritate the corneo-scleral surface for a long time. Therefore any animal showing epiphora should be carefully examined for FBs inside both conjunctival fornix and around nictitating membrane.

Ease of removal of FBs depends upon their lodgement site. Non-penetrating FBs can be easily picked up by forceps; whereas, FBs penetrating cornea or other internal structures should be handled very carefully. Attempts to retrieve penetrating ocular FBs should be done only under GA. The FBs may get broken with rough manipulation and complicate further retrieval. Damage to surrounding structures should also be minimized during such manipulations; the iris in particular is prone to haemorrhage.

Traumatic Ocular Proptosis

It refers to forward displacement of eyeball following usually a blunt trauma, bite wounds and forceful restraint. It is common in dogs and more common in brachycephalic breeds as they have shallow orbital cavity and large palpebral fissure.

Once it occurs, the palpebral margins are generally entrapped behind the eye and the contracture and continuous spasms of the orbicularis muscle prevent the

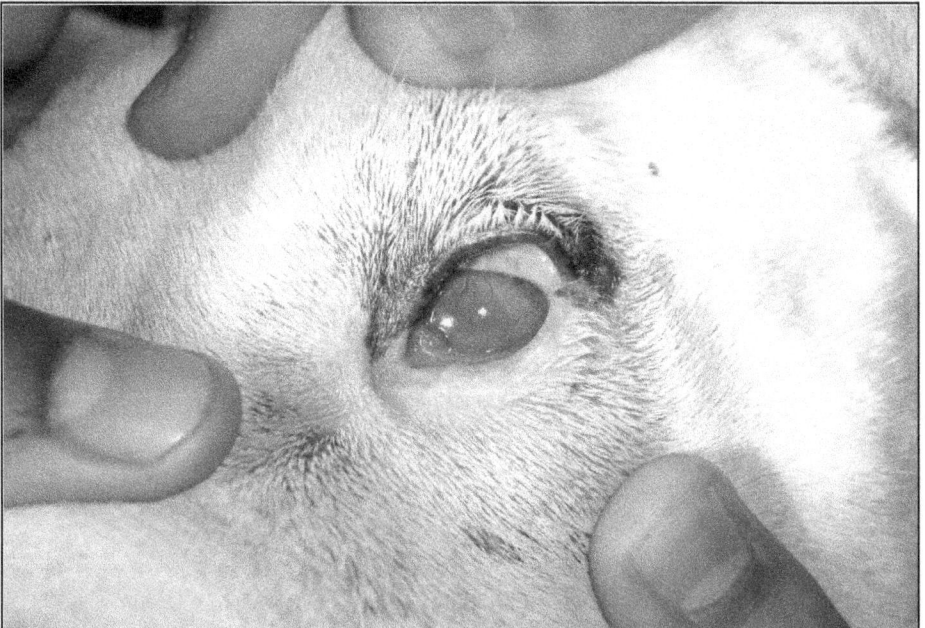

Figure 9.11: Severe Kerato-Conjuctivitis in a Dog.

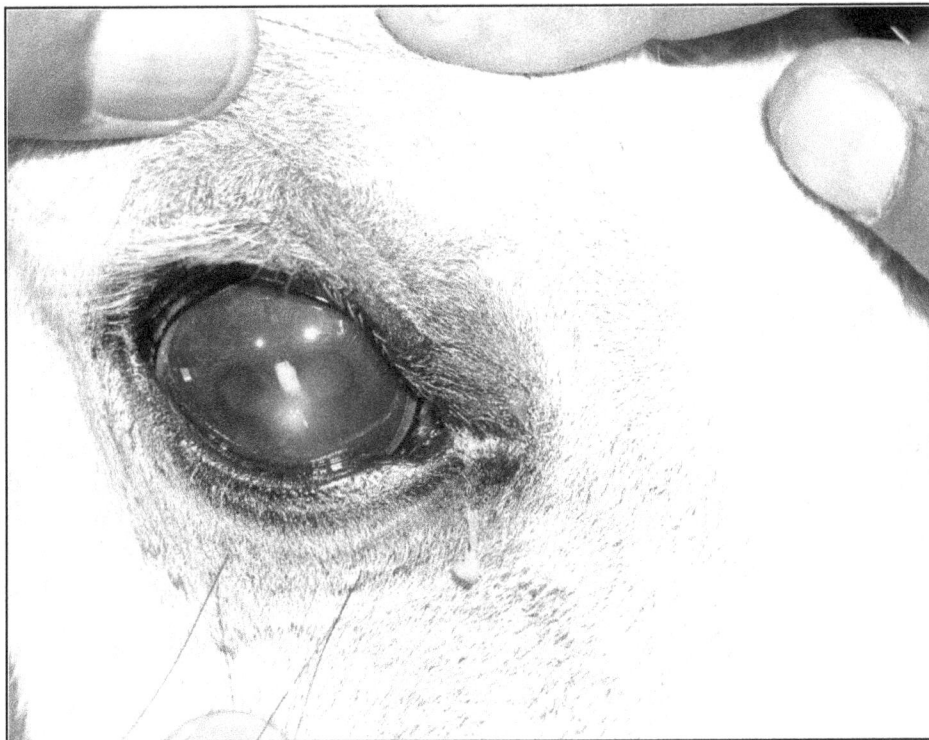

Figure 9.12: A Piece of Wheat Straw Penetrating Cornea Iris and Lens in a Cow.

eyeball to relocate to its normal position spontaneously. Ocular muscle damage, venostasis, chemosis, subconjunctival haemorrhage and corneal drying soon follow.

This condition is a surgical emergency and should be treated immediately to improve chances of restoration of vision and the shape of eye. If the eyeball is not ruptured and cornea and extra-ocular area are not much damaged, the eyeball should be replaced back surgically to its normal location. For this keep the eye moist with a BSS until the animal is anaesthetized. Lubricate the eye thoroughly with antibiotic ointment or artificial tears. Administer large doses of intravenous corticosteroids frequently (Methylprednisolone sodium succinate @ 30 mg/kg initially followed by 15 mg/g at 2 and 6 hours) to treat or prevent optic neuropathy and orbital oedema. Quickly prepare the area and induce GA with a short acting anaesthetic.

Evert and retract eyelids with the help of ophthalmic muscle hooks, and apply gentle retrograde pressure on the globe with any flat instrument or simply with moistened cotton ball to replace it; perform lateral canthotomy if required (A &C). Flush the conjunctival fornix with BSS and perform temporary tarsorrhaphy (D). The eyeball may still appear partially prolapsed and larger than normal due to venocongestion and partial filling of retrobulbar space by blood. This will improve later. If canthotomy was performed, closed it now with simple interrupted non-absorbable 4-0 sutures.

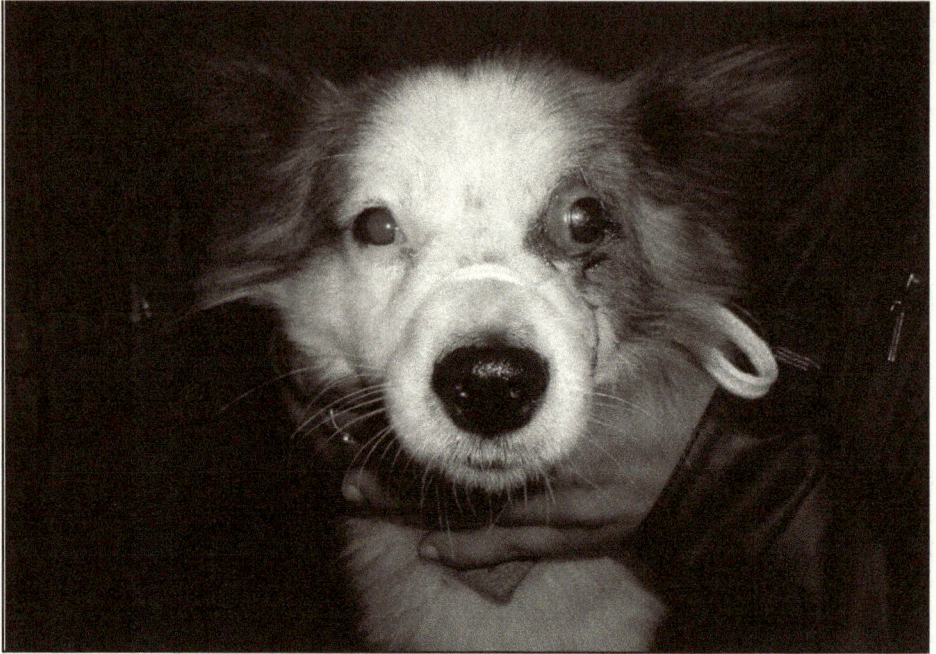

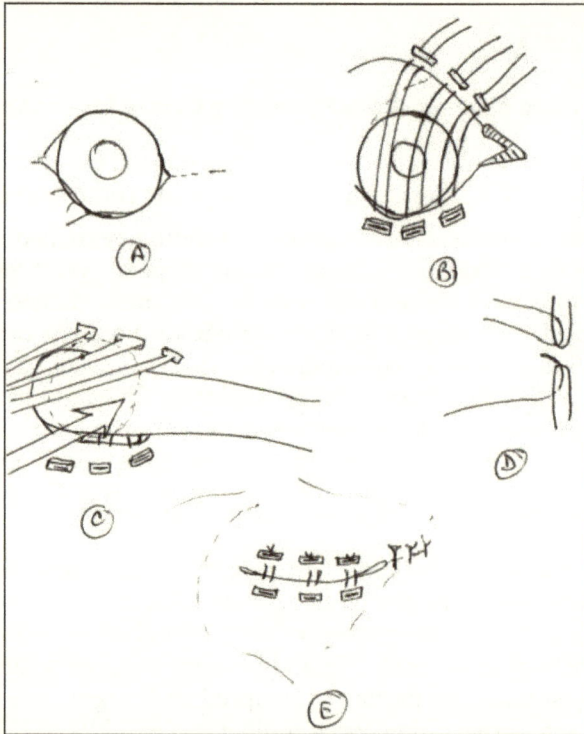

Figure 9.13: Traumatic Proptosis in a Dog and its Surgical Correction Technique.

For tarsorrhaphy, 4-0 to 5-0 non-abosorbable sutures are used in dogs. Horizontal mattress sutures are preplaced at the lid margins to appose them later. Stents are used to distribute the tension on the suture line (B). The bite of suture needle is taken only in the outer one third of the eyelid to avoid contact of sutures with cornea (D); the needle exits through the orifices of tarsal glands from eyelid margins. The sutures are tightened simultaneously and the eyelids are apposed.

Post-operatively broad spectrum systemic antibiotic is administered two to three times a day for 7-10 days. Oral prednisolone @ 1mg/kg are given for first 7

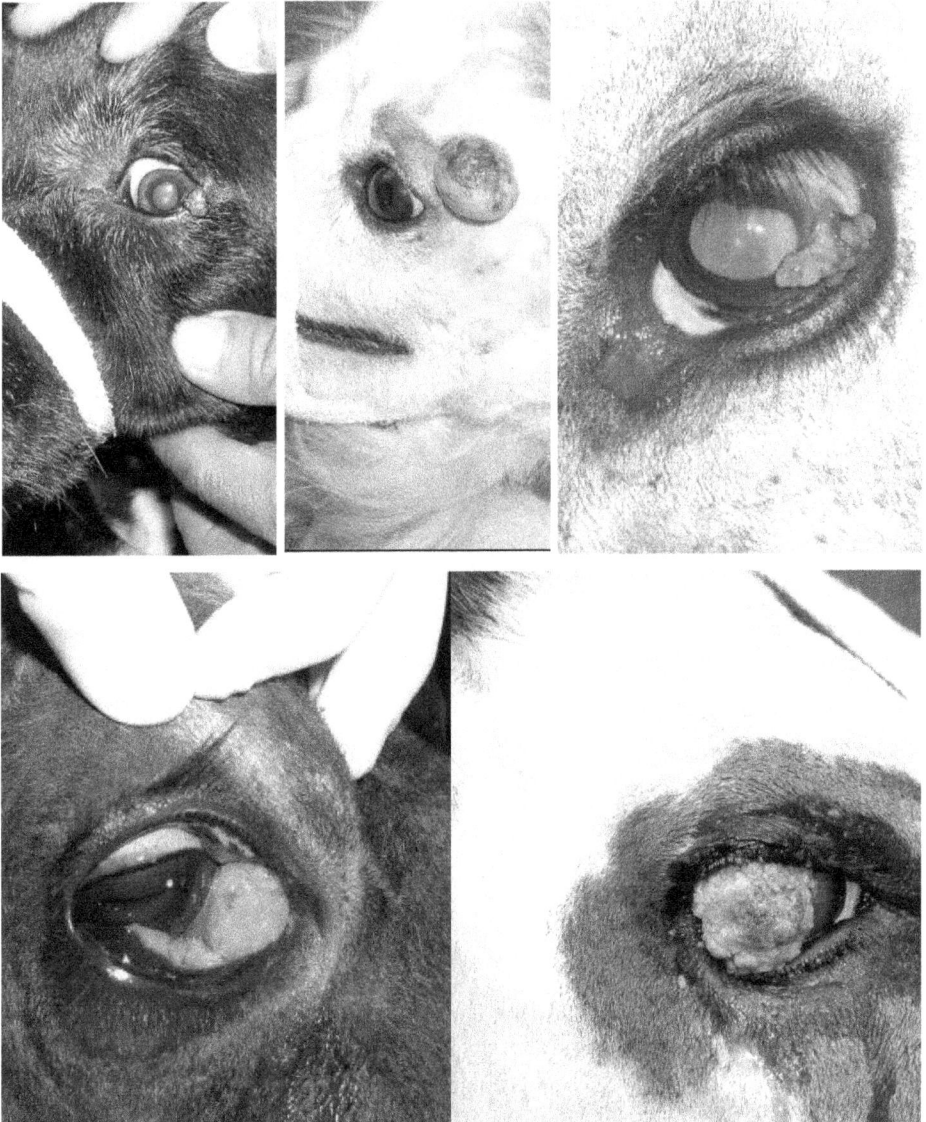

Figure 9.14: Tumours involving Eyelid, Periocular Tissue, Selura, Nictitating Membrane and Cornea in Animals.

days with decreasing doses over the next 14 days. Topical antibiotic-steroid combination and cycloplegic drug (*e.g.* 1 per cent Tropicamide) are given for 7-10 days. Cold compresses on the affected eye for the first 2-3 days and warm compresses for next 2-3 days also help in improving the condition. Elizabethan collar should be applied to prevent self-mutilation. Canthotomy sutures are to be removed after 10-14 days and tarsorrhaphy sutures after 14-28 days depending upon the condition.

Ocular Tumours

Various types of benign and malignant ocular tumours may be found in all species of animals involving different parts of the eye. Only benign types are amenable to surgical excision. These can be excised following standard operative procedure just as any other tumour.

Basic Ophthalmic Surgery Pack for Small Animals

☆	Backhaus towel clamp	6 small sized
☆	Metzenbaum scissors straight	1 small sized
☆	Metzenbaum scissors curved	1 small sized
☆	Halstead artery forceps	2 each curved and straight small sized
☆	Barraquer wire eyelid speculum	1 each small, medium and large
☆	Labermann speculum	1 small and medium size each
☆	Steven's tenotomy scissors (blunt tips)	1 each straight and curved
☆	Corneoscleral scissors Castroviejo	1 right/left pair
☆	Iris scissors	1
☆	Adson tissue forceps 1X2 teeth straight	1 small sized
☆	Entropion/chalazion forceps	1
☆	Cilia forceps	1
☆	Bishop-Harmon tissue forceps 1X2 teeth	1
☆	Bishop-Harmon tissue forceps serrated	1
☆	Lid plate	1
☆	Beaver scalpel handle	1
☆	Blade No. 6400, 6500, 6700	Q.S.
☆	Castroviejo needle holder	1
☆	Tying forceps smooth edge	Straight and curved
☆	Tying forceps serrated edge	Straight and curved
☆	Microsurgery needle holder	1
☆	Muscle hook	

☆	Silicon bulb and canula	1
☆	Cannula 18-27 G	5 different gauge
☆	SS cup/bowl	1
☆	Sterilization trays with silicon pad	1 each large size and double decker type

Miscellaneous Basic Ophthalmic Items

☆	Disposable ophthalmic cautery	1
☆	Schiotz tonometer	1
☆	Direct ophthalmoscope	1
☆	Fluorescein test strips pack	Q.S.
☆	Schirmer tear test strips pack	Q.S.
☆	Absorbable synthetic (Vicryl) suture 6-0, 8-0	Q.S.
☆	Non absorbable synthetic (Prolene/Nylon) suture 4-0, 5-0, 6-0, 8-0	Q.S.
☆	Inj. 2 per cent Hydroxypropylmethyl cellulose (Miosol-PFS)	Q.S.
☆	Eye drops 1 per cent Tropicamide (Triocyl) 2 per cent Pilocarpine (Pilocar) 0.03 per cent Flurbiprofen sod. (Flur) 0.3 per cent Hydroxypropylmethyl cellulose (Miosol) Ofloxacin-Dexamethasone (Ocipred) Gatifloxacin-Prednisolone (Gatiquin-P)	Q.S.
☆	Small torch	1
☆	Spray bottle 500 ml	2
☆	Unbreakable plastic trays	5
☆	Ear buds pack	1

10

Tracheostomy and Oesophagotomy in Cattle

Ajay Kumar Gupta

TRACHEOSTOMY

Tracheostomy refers to the surgical creation of an opening into the trachea, whereas the term tracheotomy refers to an incision in the trachea. Many surgeons use these terms virtually interchangeably.

Indications

Tracheostomy may be an emergency procedure in a situation of upper airway obstruction (due to snake bite, abscess of regional lymph node, nasopharyngeal neoplasia etc.) or an elective procedure (following nasal surgery, during laryngeal surgery, intraoral surgery or whenever post-operative respiratory obstruction is anticipated).

Surgical Anatomy

The trachea or the wind pipe is partly cartilagenous and partly membranous tube that extends from larynx along the neck to the base of the heart, where it divides into the right and the left bronchi. It also gives off the apical bronchus at the level of 3rd rib to the right lung. Trachea is kept permanently open by about 45-50 incomplete cartilagenous rings enclosed and interconnected by fibroelastic membrane that constitutes the tracheal annular ligament. The cartilagenous rings are completed dorsally by the trachealis muscle and membrana transversa. Behind the 5th ring the ends of cartilages meet dorsally producing a ridged condition.

Cervical part of trachea occupies the median position on ventral aspect of the neck and is covered ventrally by the paired sternothyrohyoideus muscle throughout its length and paired sternocephalicus muscle in the lower third of the neck. Dorsally it is related to the longus coli muscle and oesophagus, and laterally to the common carotid arteries, vagosympathetic trunk, internal jugular vein, recurrent laryngeal nerves, tracheal lymphatic trunk and deep cervical lymphnodes. The blood supply to the trachea is through the branches of the common carotid arteries and the veins go mainly to the jugular veins. The nerve supply is from the vagosympathetic trunk.

Anaesthesia and Control

In large animals sedation and/or local anaesthetic infiltration at the site are commonly used and the procedure is performed in lateral recumbency or in standing position.

Site of Incision

Mid ventral aspect at the junction of the middle and upper thirds of the neck.

Surgical Procedure

If time and airway status allow, the ventral cervical site is clipped, aseptically prepared, and infiltrated with local anaesthetic. If this is not possible, all priorities should be directed at opening the tracheal airway. A 7-10 cm midline skin incision is made at the site where the trachea is most easily palpated (junction of the middle and cranial thirds of the cervical trachea). The paired sternothyroideus and sternohyoideus muscles have a midline raphe. The ideal incision should part the musculature on the midline to expose the ventral aspect of the trachea. The incision is extended bluntly by separating the sternothyrohyoideus muscles with scissors. With a surgical blade, the membrane between the two tracheal rings is incised, parallel to the tracheal rings, over approximately one third of its circumference. The tracheostomy tube of appropriate size is inserted and secured in place with one loop of suture on either side of the tracheostomy tube. Another method is to remove an elliptical piece of cartilage from each of the two adjacent rings. A semicircular piece of cartilage is excised from the cranial surface of one ring and the caudal surface of the next ring.

For ***permanent tracheostomy*** a more extensive exposure is required as all local musculature, excessive skin, and portions of 3-4 tracheal rings are excised. After incising the skin, a section of strap muscles (sternothyroid and sternohyoid muscles) is removed, followed by removal of one-fourth to one third of the tracheal circumference from each cartilage ring. The mucosa should be preserved and incised on the midline. Enough skin should be excised to prevent loose skin from occluding the tracheostomy site. The tracheal mucosa is sutured to the skin to produce the desired stoma.

Post-operative Care

After surgery, the tracheostomy tube is removed and cleaned daily or more frequently if substantial volumes of exudate and debris accumulate in and around

Figure 10.1: Tracheostomy

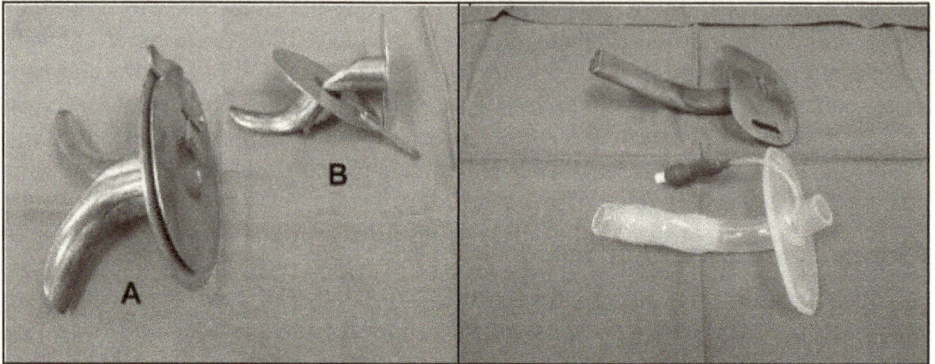

Various Types of Tracheostomy Tubes

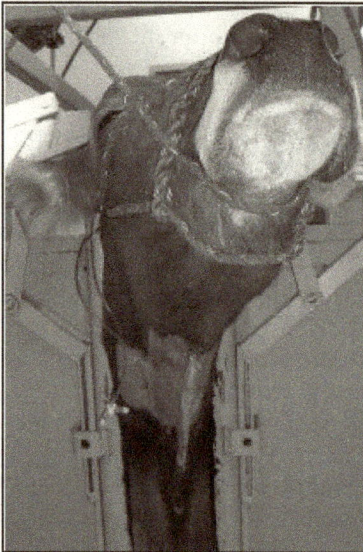

Head position for performing a tracheotomy in standing animal

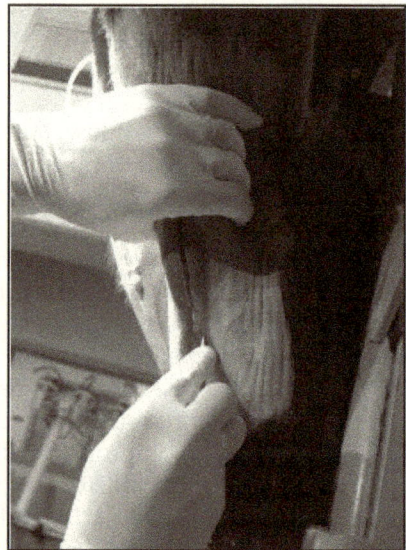

Exposing trachea after splitting the medial raphe uniting the paired sternohyoideus and sternothyroideus muscles

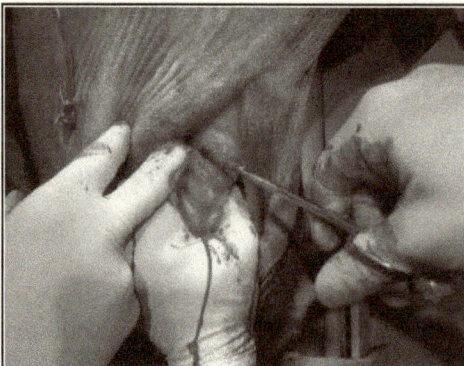

Incision of the annular ligament (Less than one half of the circumference)

Figure 10.1–*Contd...*

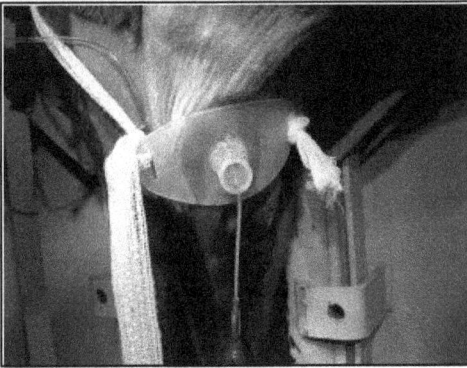

Tracheostomy tube held by a neck tie

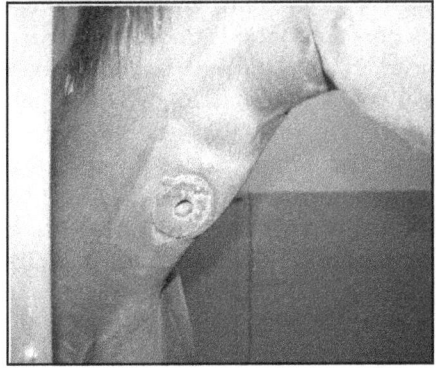

Self retaining trcheostomy tube in place in a horse

the tube's lumen. The tracheostomy site is cleaned with normal saline solution and all secretions removed during each cleaning. Petroleum jelly/oil based antibiotic cream is liberally applied at the tracheostomy site to prevent scalding by tracheal secretions. Systemic antibiotic and anti-inflammatory therapy is also indicated. The tube is removed once the primary respiratory obstruction is resolved, and the tracheostomy site is allowed to heal by second intention.

Complications

Infection is the likely complication, if attention is not paid to post-operative cleaning of tracheostomy tube and tracheostomy site. Emphysema of subcutaneous tissue can develop if air leaks along the fascial planes, but is self limiting. Tracheotomy stenosis, due to formation of excessive amounts of granulation tissue, is the potential complication and depends on the length of time the tracheostomy tube is left in place and the width of incision.

OESOPHAGOTOMY

Indications

Oesophageal obstruction, oesophageal diverticulum, oesophageal stenosis, oesophageal neoplasia etc. are the common indications of oesophagotomy.

Surgical Anatomy

The bovine oesophagus (Gullet) is 75-105 cm long musculo-membranous cylindrical tube, divided into cervical and thoracic parts, extending from the pharynx to the cardia. Because the rumen is closely related to the diaphragm, no appreciable intraabdominal portion of the oesophagus exists. Cervical oesophagus begins at pharynx in the median line and passes backwards and downwards on the dorsal surface of trachea till about the level of 3rd or 4th cervical vertebrae. At this level it crosses the trachea obliquely placing itself along the left side up to the thoracic inlet. The thoracic part begins at the level of 1st rib, continues up to 2nd or 3rd thoracic vertebrae, where it again crosses the left face of trachea obliquely upwards to gain its dorsal surface. It courses in the mediastinum, passing dorsal to the base of the heart and tracheal bifurcation. The oesophagus crosses the aortic arch and continues caudally through the oesophageal hiatus at the level of the eighth or ninth intercostal space. Structures that accompany the cervical oesophagus include the trachea and recurrent laryngeal nerve ventromedially, longus coli muscle dorsally, tracheal lymphatic trunk, deep cervical lymph nodes and carotid sheath containing common carotid artery, vagosympathetic trunk, internal jugular vein laterally. In the caudal mediastinum, the oesophagus is adjacent to the dorsal and ventral trunks of the vagus nerve. Dorsally, it is in proximity to the large caudal mediastinal lymph nodes. The oesophagus comprises of four layers that include the outer adventitial layer, muscular layers, submucosa and a thick mucosal layer that is thrown into longitudinal folds when empty. In the thoracic oesophagus the adventitial layer is replaced by a serosal covering, which is formed by the mediastinal pleura. In ruminants, except at the cranial and caudal ends, the tunica muscularis comprises the outer and inner spiral layers of striated muscle fibers that run throughout the length of the oesophagus. At the cranial and caudal ends, the inner muscle layer consists of circular fibers, whereas the outer layer consists of longitudinal fibers. Blood supply is from the cranial thyroid, common carotid and bronchoesophageal arteries. Nerve supply is from the branches of the vagus, sympathetic and recurrent laryngeal nerves.

Anaesthesia and Control

Sedation and local infiltration at the site is sometimes adequate for cervical oesophagotomy in standing position or right lateral recumbency. General anaesthesia and positive pressure ventilation are essential for a thoracic oesophagotomy.

Site of Incision

The incision site is along the superior or inferior border of jugular furrow close to the level of obstruction on the left side of the neck for cervical oesophagotomy. A left-sided rib resection is usually performed for the thoracic oesophagotomy.

Surgical Procedure

A lateral or ventrolateral approach is typically described for performing a cervical oesophagotomy. As the oesophagus is normally a flaccid tube that is difficult to recognise among the cervical muscles, it must be made visible by inserting a stomach tube up to the level of the obstruction prior to anaesthesia. The neck is prepared for aseptic surgery. An incision about 3-4 inches long is made along the superior or inferior border of left jugular furrow cutting through the skin and cervical cutaneous fascia. The oesophagus can be approached either between the trachea and sternocephalicus muscle, or between this muscle and the jugular vein. The oesophagus is recognized by its characteristic pink colour. The affected area is isolated from the surgical field using moist sponges. The wall of the oesophagus is

Figure 10.2: Oesophagotomy

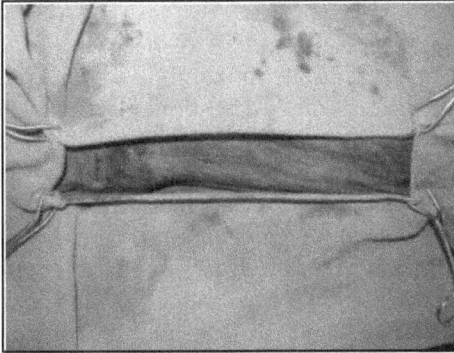

Left jugular groove aseptically prepared
for oesophagotomy

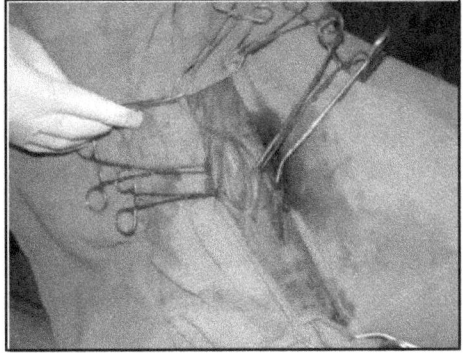

Oesophagus exposed by retracting
sternocephalicus muscle dorsally

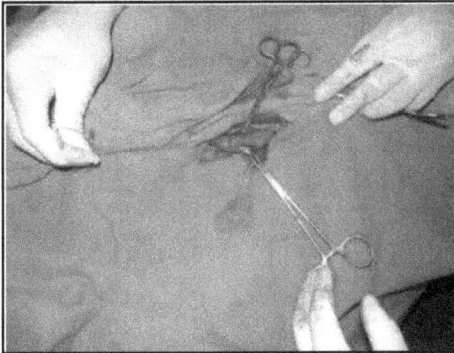

Longitudinal incision on oesophagus

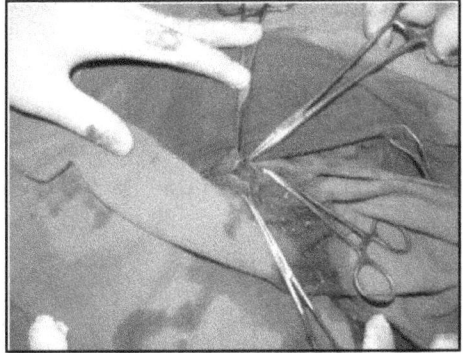

First layer oesophageal suturing using
simple interrupted sutures with knots
inside the lumen

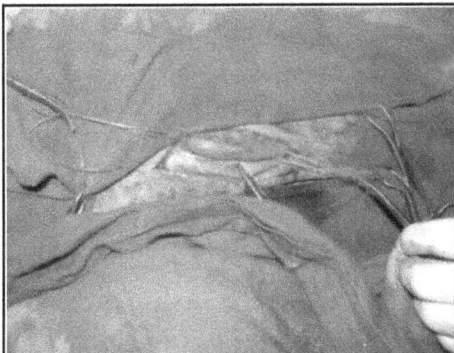

Second layer oesophageal suturing
using simple continuous pattern

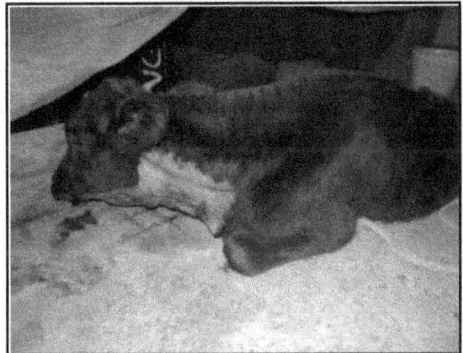

Oesophagotomy completed

incised longitudinally over the desired length cranial or caudal to the obstruction to get into the lumen and the obstruction is relieved.

Primary closure is recommended if the oesophageal wall has a normal appearance. If considerable dead space exists, a closed suction drain is advised for the first 48-72 hours. If the oesophageal wall is compromised, it should be allowed to heal by second intention with daily wound care. Primary oesophageal closure involves a 2-layer technique. The mucosa and submucosa are closed together in either a simple continuous or simple interrupted pattern. A synthetic absorbable (*e.g.*, polyglactin-910, polydioxanone or polyglyconate) suture material is preferred. It is recommended the knots be tied within the oesophageal lumen to prevent contamination of the wound by ingesta migrating along suture tracts. The muscular layer can be closed by using either an absorbable or nonabsorbable noncapillary suture with a simple interrupted or mattress pattern. Skin is closed in a routine manner.

Post-operative Care

Food and water are withheld and adequate fluid therapy is given for several days; and soft foods must follow until healing is complete. Proper wound care, a course of antibiotics and anti-inflammatory medication is recommended.

Complications

Possible complications include wound dehiscence resulting in fistula, and stenosis of oesophagus due to scar formation.

Special Considerations

Unfortunately, oesophageal surgery in any species is fraught with complications. Most of the oesophagus does not have a serosal covering, which is important in forming a fibrin seal. Furthermore, the esophageal lumen is not clean; constant movement occurs during swallowing, and its location causes tension on any suture line. The proximity of the recurrent laryngeal nerve to the oesophagus can have deleterious effects on manipulations. Once the muscular coat is incised, the oesophagus separates into two layers: the elastic inner layer, which is composed of mucosa and submucosa, and the outer muscular layer and adventitia. The inner layer provides the greatest tensile strength during oesophageal closure. Preservation of blood supply, aseptic technique, apposition of tissues without tension, and appropriate perioperative management are essential for a successful outcome.

11

Foreign Body Syndrome in Bovines

R.N. Chaudhary

Ingestion of foreign bodies by large ruminants causes a variety of problems in digestive system. Previously, foreign body syndrome (FBS) was synonymous to traumatic reticuloperitonitis (TRP). However, in the present era, when non-degradable plastic is being extensively used, it is a common foreign material to be ingested by bovines (mainly stray cattle). There are two types of foreign bodies often ingested by bovines - potential and non-potential. Potential foreign bodies (like wire, nail, needle or any other sharp stiff metallic/non-metallic object which is able to penetrate the GIT) cause TRP and its associated complications. However, non-potential foreign bodies (polythene bags, rope pieces, cloth pieces etc.) mainly cause either impaction of rumen or obstruction of rumeno-reticular orifice, popularly called as plastic menace in cattle.

The problem of FBS in bovines arises because of indifferent manners of prehension, little mastication and peculiar arrangement of gastric apparatus. Lack of grazing land and the practice of intensive management have led to increasing tendency of maintaining large ruminants under stable condition, and on dry feed for longer period during the year. This, coupled with mechanization of agriculture and consequent increase in the metallic debris in the feed and fodder, seems to increase the occurrence of TRP each year. Adult dairy cattle and buffaloes are most commonly affected because of their longer exposure to foreign materials with age. In India, incidence of TRP appears to be higher in buffaloes than in cattle, however, polythene menace is higher in cattle than in buffaloes.

Pathogenesis

Once a potential foreign body reaches the fore-stomach, it lodges in the honeycomb of the reticulum. The vigorous contractions of the reticulum aided by the movement of diaphragm make thin sharp hard objects to penetrate through the reticular wall. The most common sites of penetration include antero-ventral wall, ventral wall or anterior wall of the reticulum. The number of lesions is directly related to the number of foreign bodies. Perforation of the wall of reticulum, followed by contamination of peritoneal cavity, cause an acute local peritonitis, which may spread to cause diffuse peritonitis or remain localized to cause subsequent damage like vagal indigestion and diaphragmatic hernia. Penetrating foreign bodies may proceed beyond peritoneum and damage other organs causing several complications *viz.* reticular abscess, reticular fistula, diaphragmatic hernia, diaphragmatic abscess, traumatic pericarditis (TP), traumatic sternebrae, pyothorax, abscessation of liver and spleen, traumatic pneumonia and pleurisy.

The inflammatory changes in the peritoneal cavity lead to formation of adhesions, which play an important role in causing symptoms of inappetance to anorexia. Extensive adhesions of reticulum and/or rumen with diaphragm and other organs like abdominal wall might interfere with their contraction, eructation process and the outflow of ingesta to the lower digestive tract. Due to digestive disorders and inappetance for many days, the metabolic profile of such animals is likely to be compromised.

Non-potential foreign bodies like nuts, coins and stones lie harmlessly and may be passed out in the faeces. However, the materials like plastics, cloths, ropes, leather pieces get accumulated in the rumeno-reticulum. The movement of the fore-stomach churns these materials and a very hard space occupying bulk is formed. It occupies most of rumeno-reticular space and very less space is left for ingesta proper. The ruminal microflora is disturbed and sometime reticulo-omasal orifice may be occluded leading to cessation of faeces after a few days.

Diagnosis

Clinical Signs

A wide variation exists in the extent and intensity of clinical picture of FBS depending on the extent of injury, duration of illness, anatomical and physiological status of the organs involved and pregnancy status of the animal. Most of the animals with TRP are dull, depressed and appear stiff. The temperature and heart rate may be increased. There is rapid drop in the milk yield, anorexia, ruminal and reticular atony leading to ruminal impaction with slight tympany and absence of cudding, protrusion of neck, disinclination to lie down. Spontaneous grunting accentuated by movement, defaecation, micturation and becomes very marked on pinching withers or applying pressure to xiphisternal region. Such animals have abducted elbows with the hind limbs held more under the body. Sometimes, trembling of muscles over left side on the back of elbow, occasionally over the rumen and rarely on both sides is noticed. In chronic peritonitis, there is repeated attacks of indigestion or reduced milk production. The tension of abdominal muscles leads to 'gaunt' or

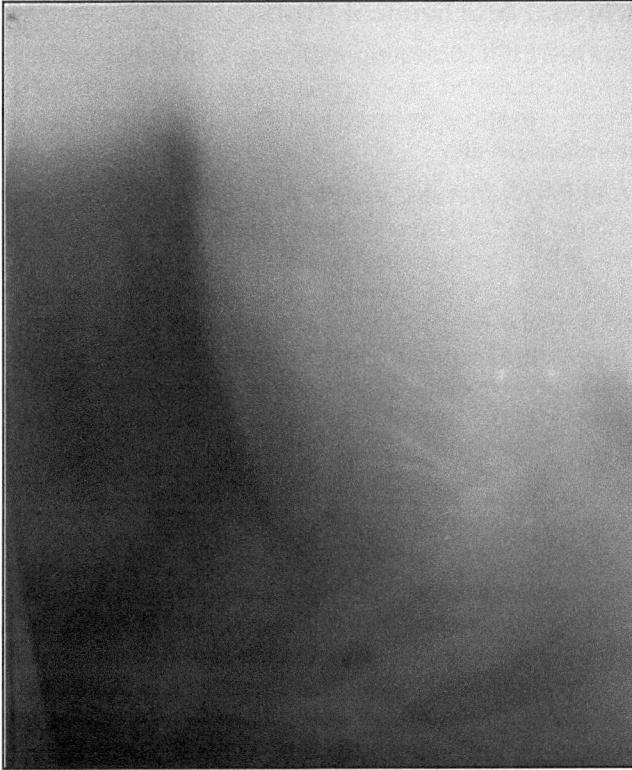

Figure 11.1: Radiograph Showing Potential Foreign Bodies in the Reticulum.

'tucked up' appearance. Symptoms like short stepping and rarely, crouching and kicking at the belly may also occur.

The animal suffering from plastic menace is usually weak, anaemic, debilitated and sometime recumbent when reported for the treatment. There is no history of fever. Animal passes scanty faeces with straining. On abdominal palpation, rumen is hard, impacted and can not be pressed even with fist.

Radiography and Ultrasonography

A plain radiograph of the reticular area is the best tool to diagnose TRP. Good quality radiographs of diagnostic value are easily obtained preferably in lateral recumbency. Radiograph of reticular region obtained in standing position may not be of much diagnostic value.

A healthy bovine reticulum appears ultrasonographically as a half-moon shaped structure with a smooth contour that contract at regular intervals. When relaxed, the reticulum is situated immediately adjacent to the diaphragm and ventral abdominal wall. The reticular contents are partly gaseous, so cannot be seen on ultrasonogram. Both the radiography and ultrasonography are not very useful in diagnosing the FBS due to non-potential and non-metallic foreign bodies.

Hematological and Biochemical Profile

In early cases of TRP, TLC is in normal range while neutrophilia is seen with a large number of unsegmented neutrophils. In early acute diffuse peritonitis, the neutrophil-lymphocyte ratio is reversed and decreases as the lesion becomes more chronic and adhesions develop.

Cows with TRP have elevated titrable acidity in milk and increased standard bicarbonate, decreased potassium and chloride concentration in plasma. In affected animals the mean total plasma protein remains on the higher side of normal range (> 80g/L) with increase in total globulin. The plasma fibrinogen concentration is generally over 8 g/L and on gluteraldehyde test, clotting in most of the animals occurs within 6 minutes. Trypsin inhibitor concentration in blood is substantially elevated and this may be used for screening the animals showing clinical signs of TRP as either positive (> 8 g/ml) or negative.

There is reduction in pH, infusorial count, volatile fatty acids and ammonia content of the rumen fluid. The amount of peritoneal fluid is increased. The physical characteristic and cellular contents of the fluid is altered. A relatively accurate diagnosis of peritonitis can be made if the nucleated cell count is > 6000 cells/μl and a total protein concentration is > 3 g/dl. A more accurate diagnosis can be made by performing a differential cell count and if neutrophils account for > 40 per cent of the cells and eosinophils for < 10 per cent, a diagnosis of peritonitis is indicated. A variety of bacteria like *Corynebacterium pyogenes*, *Spherophorus necrophorus*, *Escherichia coli* and *Salmonella* species may be found in the localized lesions caused by perforation of the reticulum. In cases of plastic menace there will not be any marked alteration in haemato-biochemical profile of the affected animals.

Differential Diagnosis

The other diseases which present manifestation like TRP are atony of rumen or intestine, gastric/intestinal flatulence acetonemia, acute metritis and metroperitonitis, peritonitis from external trauma, lying down condition of animal due to painful feet, penetration of involuted uterus and vagina with catheter, post-operative peritonitis, perforation of abomasal ulcers, penetration of rectum by any foreign body, tubercular peritonitis, ephemeral fever, pyelonephritis, hepatic and splenic abscesses. The complete history with careful observation of clinical signs, critical examination combined with laboratory and radiographic findings help in distinguishing these diseases from TRP.

Treatment

Generally, two methods of treatment are used for TRP, conservative treatment and surgery, but combination may be used effectively. It is better to treat the animal conservatively for the first 3 days, and if marked improvement has not occurred by that time laparorumenotomy may be performed. In conservative treatment, the animal is immobilized for two weeks, no walking is permitted, front feet are elevated and broad spectrum antibiotics, analgesics and rumenotorics are administered. A fasting for initial three days may be recommended. Laparorumenotomy is the

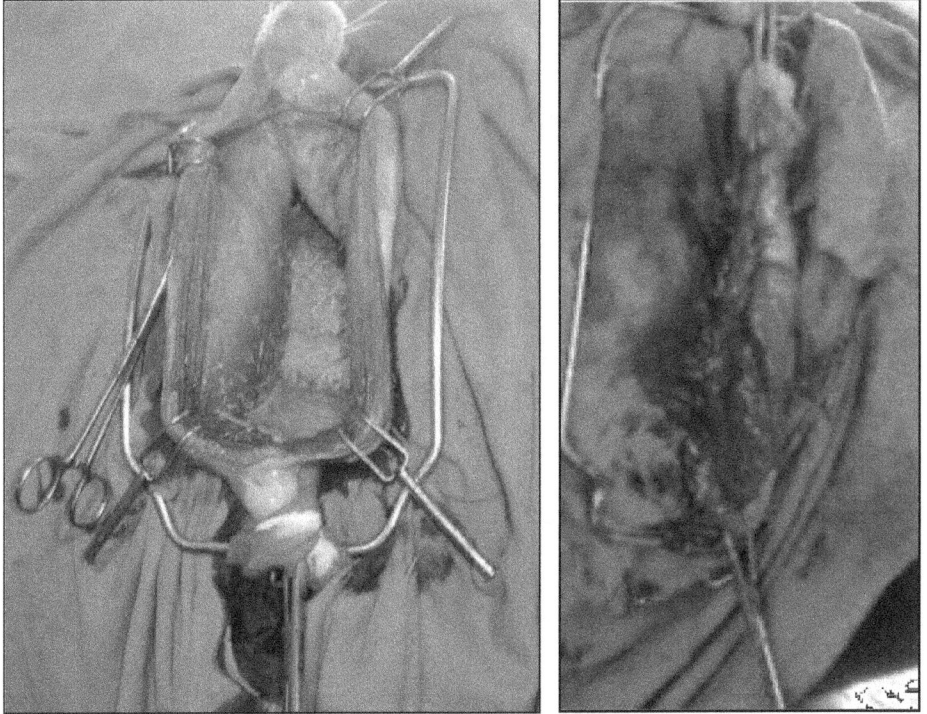

Figure 11.2: Laparorumenotomy in a Buffalo.

treatment of choice in cases of plastic menace and in animals with last trimester of pregnancy.

If the laparorumenotomy is accomplished in early phase of the disease, 100 per cent recovery is anticipated. Even reticular and perireticular abscesses, and extrareticular fibrous nodules can be treated during laparorumenotomy. Animal's health returns to normal in most of the cases.

12

Medial Patellar Desmotomy

Abhishek Chandra Saxena

Medial patellar desmotomy is a surgical incision to severe the medial patellar ligament in the animals suffering from dorsal/upward fixation of patella.

Local Names

Jhanak, Sarnail, Ragda, Tanch, Tanak.

Indications

Upward/Dorsal fixation of patella.

Etiology/Predisposing Factors

- ☆ Exploitation activity
- ☆ External trauma leading to laceration or elongation of the ligamentous structures
- ☆ Breed and genetic predisposition
- ☆ Faulty conformation of the hind limb
- ☆ Morphological changes of the medial trochlear ridge of femur
- ☆ Damage to the nerve supplying the quadriceps femoris muscle.

Symptoms

Upward fixation of patella can be unilateral or bilateral, and can be permanent or recurrent in nature. It occurs mostly in buffaloes but is also reported frequently in young working bullocks. In horses, it occurs most frequently in young ponies working on hills and in animals with a faulty conformation of the hind limbs.

Recurrent dorsal fixation is not apparent in resting animals in which the patella occupies its normal position in relation to the femoral trochlea. It is manifested during progression by an intermittent fixation of the patella through the hooking of the medial patellar ligament over the prominent upper extremity of the trochlear ridge. When the animal is forced to move, the condition becomes evident by occasional jerky steps during otherwise normal progression. It frequently disappears as the animal "warms up". In due course as the condition progresses, the symptoms become more frequent and the gait more obviously disturbed. Stifle and the hock joints are periodically fixed in extension and this gives the limb an unusual rigidity, while over-flexion of the fetlock causes the toe of the hoof to drag upon the ground during progression.

Animals suffering from permanent dorsal fixation, when forced to walk, carry their leg rigidly with the fetlock flexed and the toe dragged on the ground with the weight supported by the flexed digit. After some time, animal adapts its gait by bringing the limb forward in abduction in the swinging phase, without flexion of the hock and stifle joints. When an attempt is made to back the animal, it often refuses to move.

Clinical Examination

On clinical examination of the animals having recurrent dorsal fixation, the patella is found to be unusually mobile and in these cases it can readily be carried dorsally by slight manual pressure. If this is done and the animal is induced to move, the typical "locked" gait is seen and later, when the patella frees itself, a thudding sensation may be detected. The symptoms may be induced to appear in an exaggerated form by circling the animal with the affected limb on the inner side, while circling in the opposite direction with the affected limb outermost, lessens the symptoms.

Anatomy of Stifle Joint

Stifle joint consists of two major articulations *viz.* femoro-patellar and femoro-tibial. The femoro-patellar joint is formed between trochlea of the femur and articular surface of the patella. Patella is connected to the cranial tibial tuberosity by patellar ligaments. The patellar ligaments are medial, middle and lateral. In blind method of surgery, it is very important to identify and palpate the medial patellar ligament.

Surgical Procedure

Main aim of medial patellar desmotomy is to dislodge the patella from medial trochlear ridge, thus leading to free movement of stifle joint. Surgery can be performed with the animal in the standing position or in lateral recumbency. There are two common methods to this surgery *viz.* blind/closed method and open method.

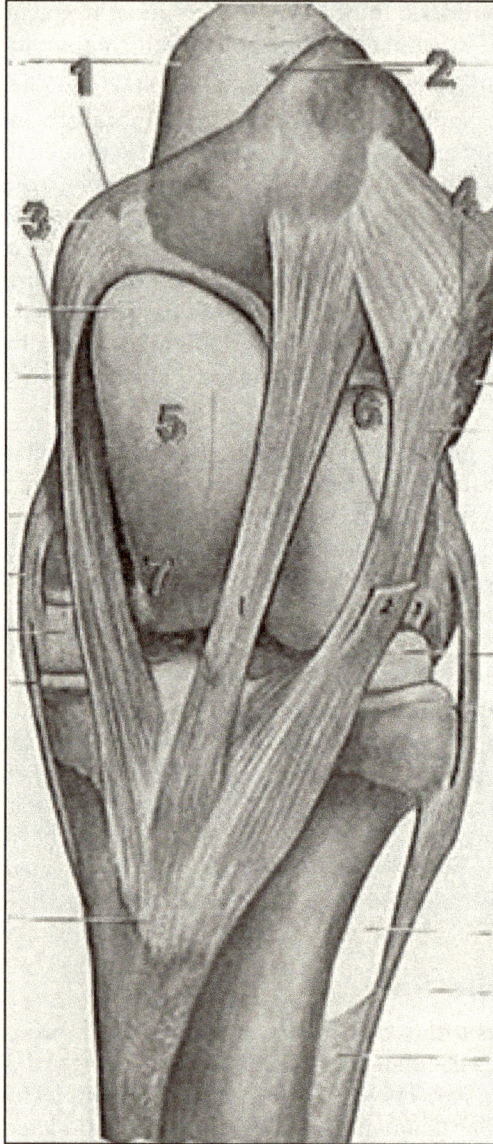

Figure 12.1: Front View of Stifle Joint.
1. Parapatellar fibrocartilage; 2. Patella; 3. Medial patellar ligament; 4. Attachment of biceps femoris; 5. Medial trochlear ridge; 6. Lateral patellar ligament; 7. Middle patellar ligament; 8. Cranial tibial tuberosity.

Standing Approach with Blind Method

The site of the skin incision is indicated by a small depression that may be felt between the middle and medial patellar ligaments above their insertion on the tibial tuberosity. The operational site is shaved and painted with tincture of iodine.

Local anaesthetic (2 per cent lignocaine, 2-5 ml) is injected subcutaneously over and around the ligament. Sterile surgical gloves are worn and the usual aseptic precautions observed. A small incision is made in the skin between the middle and medial patellar ligaments just proximal to the tibial tuberosity, taking care not to penetrate the joint capsule.

A tenotom is then pushed through the skin incision under the medial patellar ligament, near its insertion at tibial tuberosity, with its cutting edge in vertical direction. Once positioned correctly, the cutting edge is then directed towards the ligament. The tenotom is then slowly moved while strongly pressed against the ligament, which is normally transected in a single movement of the blade. Severance of the ligament is indicated by the development of a deep depression between the cut ends. If the ligament is not completely transected the procedure is repeated.

Blind Method in Lateral Recumbency

In uncooperative patients, it is difficult to perform surgery in standing condition and such animals are cast and restrained on the ground with the affected limb at lower side. Forelimbs and the upper hind limb are tied together, and the affected limb is extended backward by pulling a rope tied at the region of fetlock. Pushing the point of hock towards the ground, rotates the stifle joint to better expose the site of incision. Cranial tibial tuberosity is located and the groove between the medial

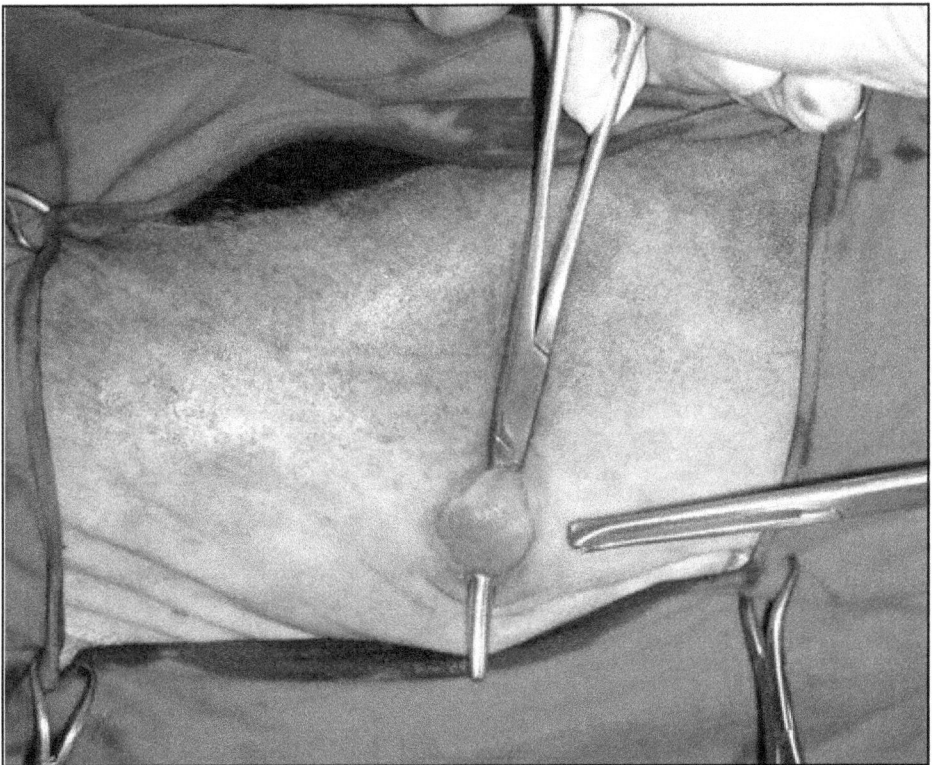

and middle patellar ligaments is then palpated. In this position, medial patellar ligament occupies the topmost position and is traced easily. Surgery is then completed in the same manner as in standing approach.

Open Method

In open method, after aseptic preparation of the surgical site on the affected limb and infiltration of local anaesthesia, a 3 cm linear incision is given 0.5 cm lateral to the medial patellar ligament near its insertion on the tibial tuberosity. Artery forceps are used for blunt dissection of the fascia from underneath the medial patellar ligament, and the ligament is then lifted over the forceps. After properly exteriorizing the ligament, it is cut transversely using a scalpel. The skin incision is closed by a few interrupted sutures.

Post-operative Care

Daily antiseptic dressing of the surgical wound and post-operative antibiotic cover, especially after open method, is all that is needed post-surgery. The results are miraculous and animal walks without a limp immediately after successful surgery.

Possible Post-operative Complications

☆ Transaction of middle patellar ligament

☆ Transaction of collateral ligaments

☆ Penetration of joint capsule

☆ Haemorrhage

☆ Infection

13

Surgical Management of Intestinal Obstruction

H.R. Bhardwaj

Intussusception is the invagination or telescoping of the one segment of bowel into the lumen of its adjacent segment and is the frequent cause of intestinal obstruction in cattle.

The intestinal obstruction implies to the failure of the intestinal contents to move in a normal aboral direction. The morbidity and mortality in intestinal obstruction cases varies considerably and depend on the type of obstruction, location of obstruction in the intestinal tract and its duration.

Etiology

Etiological factors of intestinal obstruction include conditions such as enteritis and increased peristalsis, intestinal parasitism, abrupt dietary changes, drug induced changes in intestinal motility, mural or luminal lesions, impacted food material, abscessaton, foreign bodies and tearing of mesentery and trapping of intestinal loop.

Pathophysiology

Accumulation of ingesta in higher segment of obstructed intestine results in distension of abdomen. The right side of abdomen enlarges as a result of distension of small intestine with fluid. The fluid, gas and digesta that accumulate proximal to the obstruction arise from sources including saliva, swallowed air, pancreatic and bile secretion, gas from bacterial fermentation, ingested fluid and solids and secretions from intestinal mucosa. Absorption from bowel immediately above the obstruction is hampered while secretions continued in normal amounts. Secretions accumulate in the bowel lumen and result in dehydration. Signs of early colic had been reported to be caused by tension on the mesentery from the invaginating portion of the intestine. With the passage of time, ischemia of the invaginated portion leads to loss of sensation from tension receptors.The rumen becomes distended with fluid regurgitated from abomasum.

Clinical Signs

The most important clinical signs of intestinal obstruction in cattle is scanty faeces, which often contain blood and mucous, and sausage-shaped mass may be detected upon abdominal palpation.

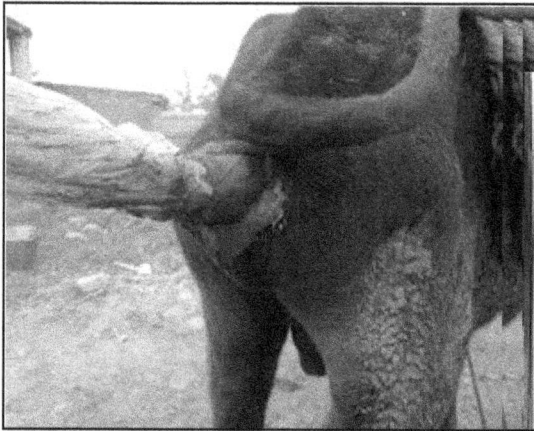

Figure 13.1: Perrectal Examination-Mucus with Tarry Colour Faeces.

The reticulo-ruminal contractions have been reported to be suppressed and may persist with reduced vigour throughout the course of disease in intestinal obstruction affected animals. History of anorexia has been reported in all the animals of different species suffering from intestinal obstructions. A cow suffering from intestinal obstruction passes no faeces. The bovines suffering from intestinal obstruction in first few hours, exhibits signs of colic characterized by violent behaviour or forceful kicking at belly with hind legs. Frequent sitting and standing up, paddling of limbs, stretching, recumbency and arching of back.

Diagnosis

Intussuscepted mass had been reported to be palpable in only minority of affected adult cattle, although, distended loops of small intestine are palpable per-rectal in 50 per cent of cases suffering with intussusception. Diagnosis is also done on the basis of clinical signs such as colicky pain, anorexia and absence of faeces. Moreover, the intestinal obstruction cases can be diagnosed on the basis clinical and laboratory findings.

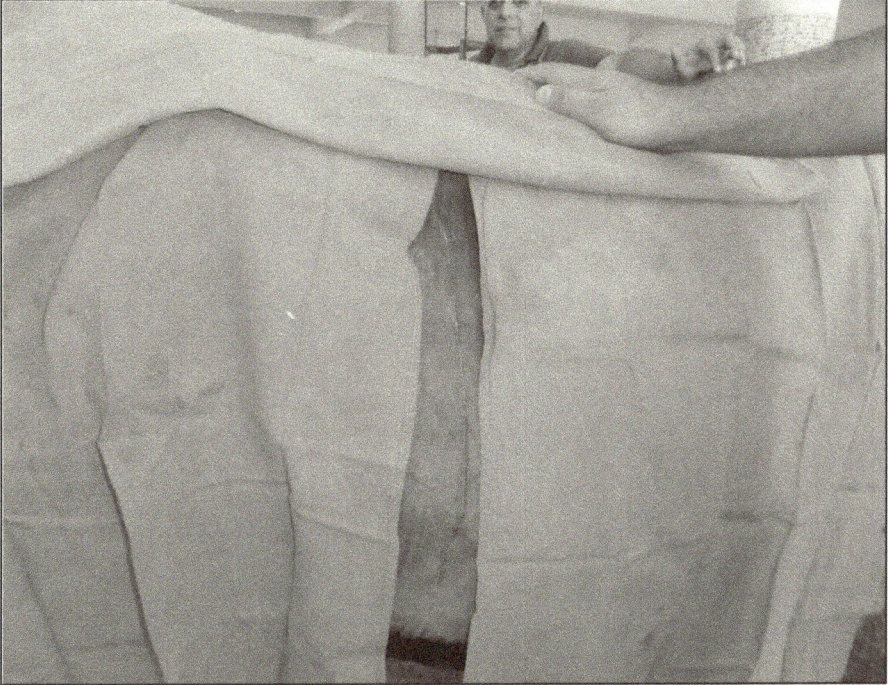

Figure 13.2: Preparation of Cow for Intestinal Surgery through Right Paralumber Fossa.

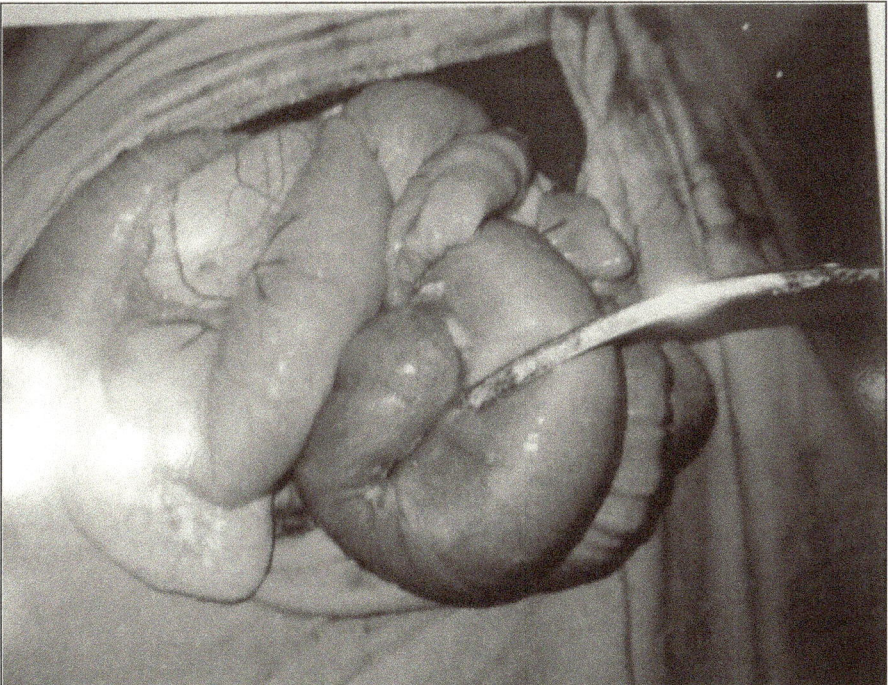

Figure 13.3: Exteriorized Obstructed Mass.

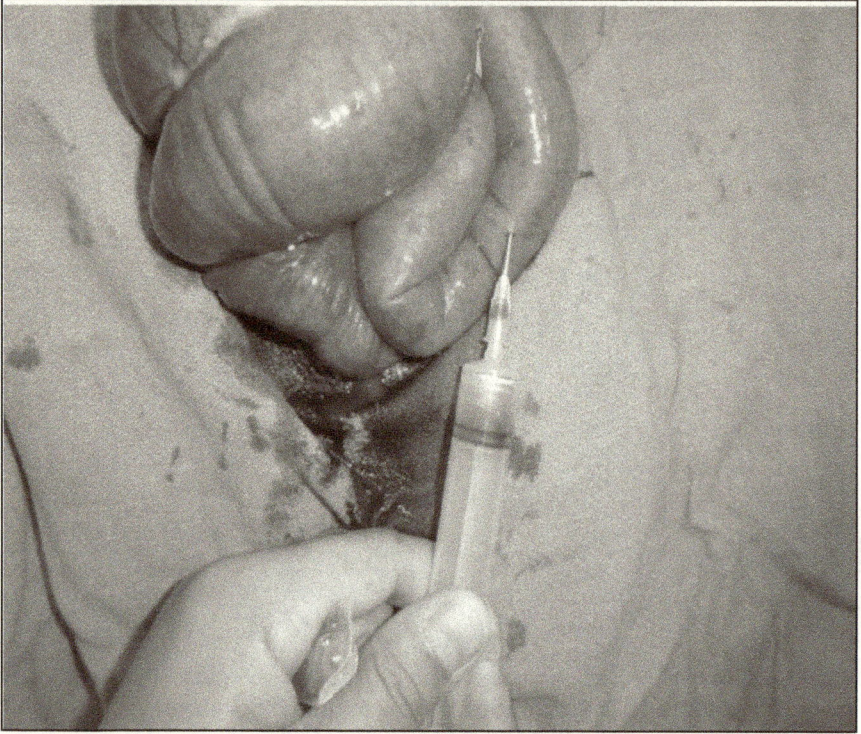

Figure 13.4: Decompression of Gas Filled Oral Part of the Intestine.

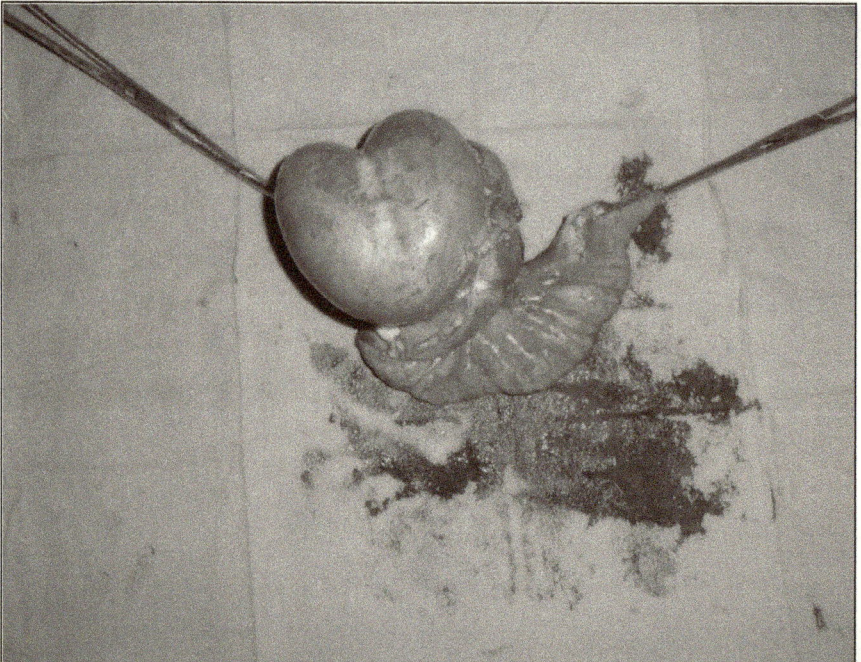

Figure 13.5: Removal of Intussuscepted Mass .

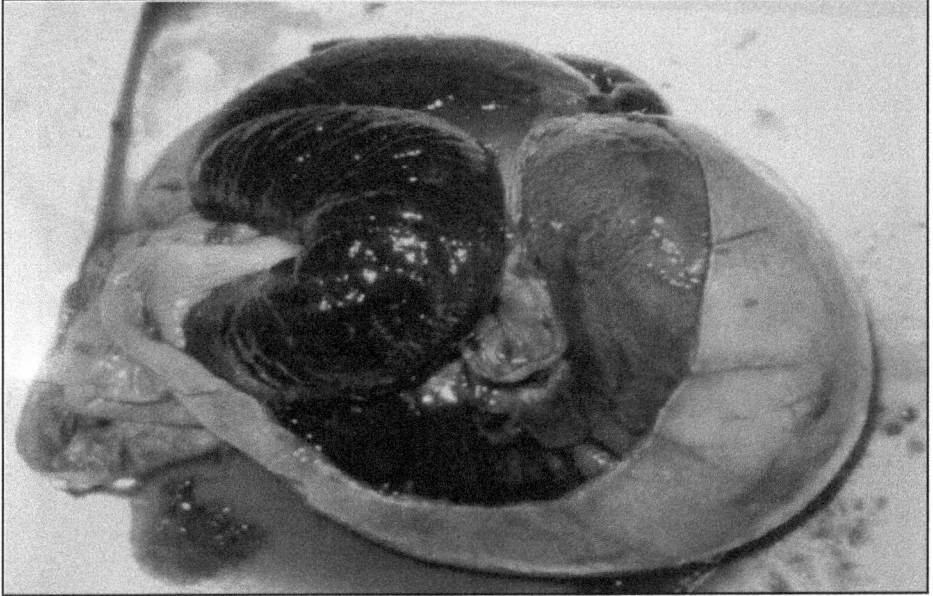

Figure 13.6: Inner Invaginated Layers after Resection which Shows Necrosis.

Surgical Treatment

Small intestinal obstructions have been reported to be repaired surgically by means of enterotomy or enterectomy, *i.e.* resection and end-to-end entero-anastomosis or side to side anastomosis. These traditional techniques have been demonstrated as time consuming and have also resulted in increased chances of anastomotic leakage; over expose the surgical site and thus cause the unnecessary trauma to increased proliferation of enteric bacteria leading, causing peritonitis, adhesions, leakage, seepage and ultimately mortality.

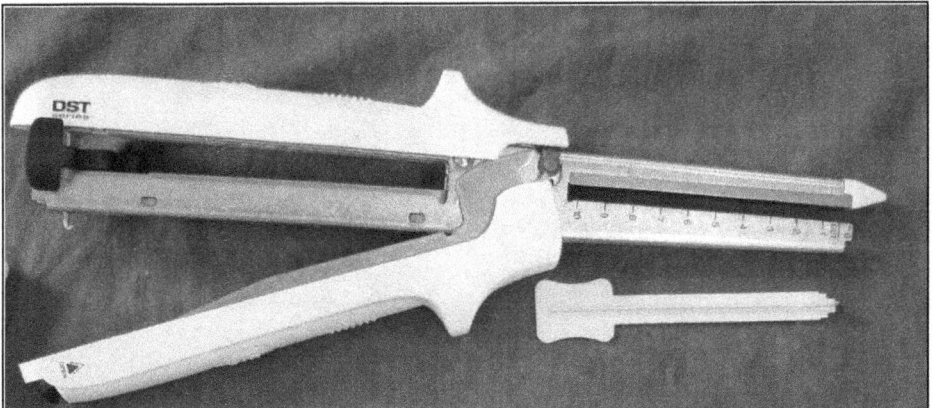

Figure 13.7: GIA Stapling Devices.

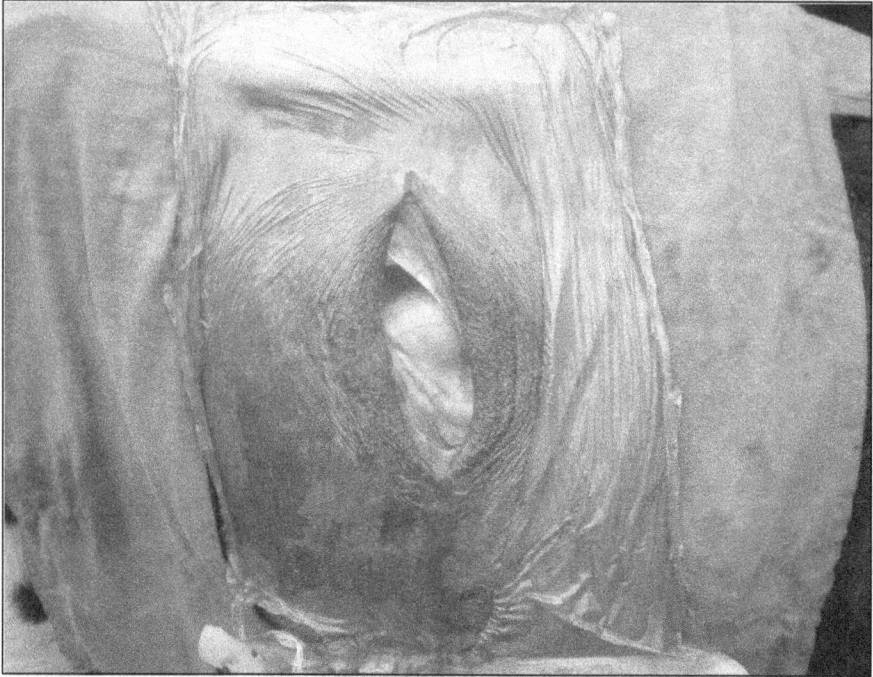

Figure 13.8: Surgical Incision at Right Flank to Approach Abdomen.

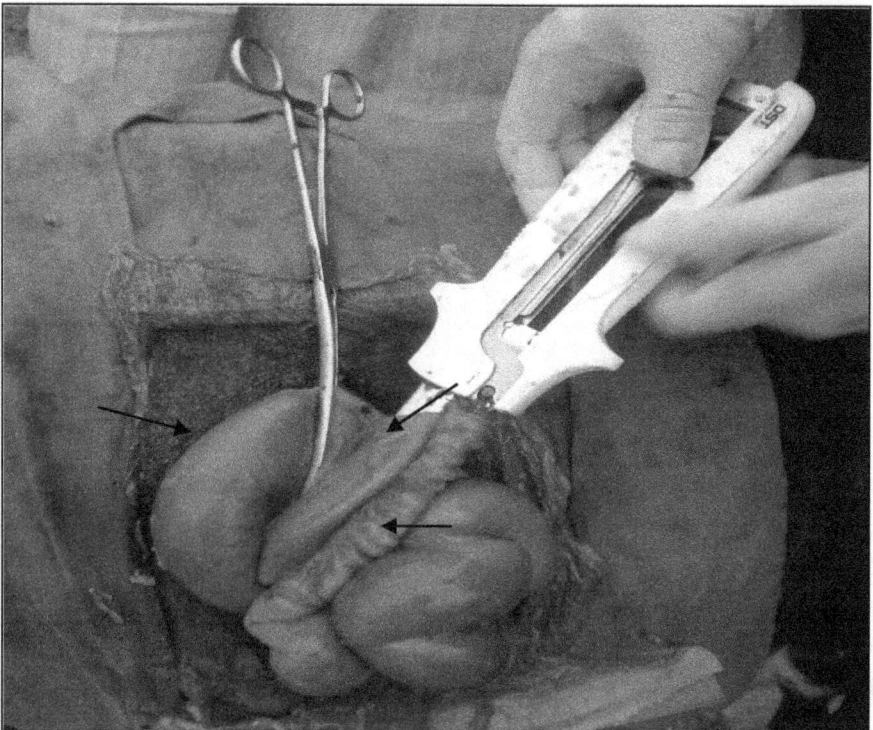

Figure 13.9: Insertion, Locking and Firing and Sectioning with GIA Stapling Device.

Recently, stapling technique has been demonstrated as better technique and can be used at field level as it consumes less time in construction of anastomosis, causes less tissue trauma and prevents prolonged exposure of surgical site to the environment. Moreover, we have bypassed intussuscepted mass in treatment of intussusception. The main advantage of bypass intussusception anastomosis using stapler is reduced risk of mesenteric bleeding. The other advantages of use of stapling devices for entero-anastomosis include short surgical time, less tissue trauma, least intra-operative contamination, protection of vasculatures and eventually early restoration.

Intussusception Bypass Surgery

Intussuscepted part of the intestine is exteriorized through the incision on the right flank. The parts oral and aboral to the intussusception are identified and small nick incisions are made on both these parts.

The limbs of the stapler are withdrawn after joining the bowel segments and double staggered anastomotic staple lines surrounding the created stoma. The nick incisions are closed with 1-0 chromic catgut.

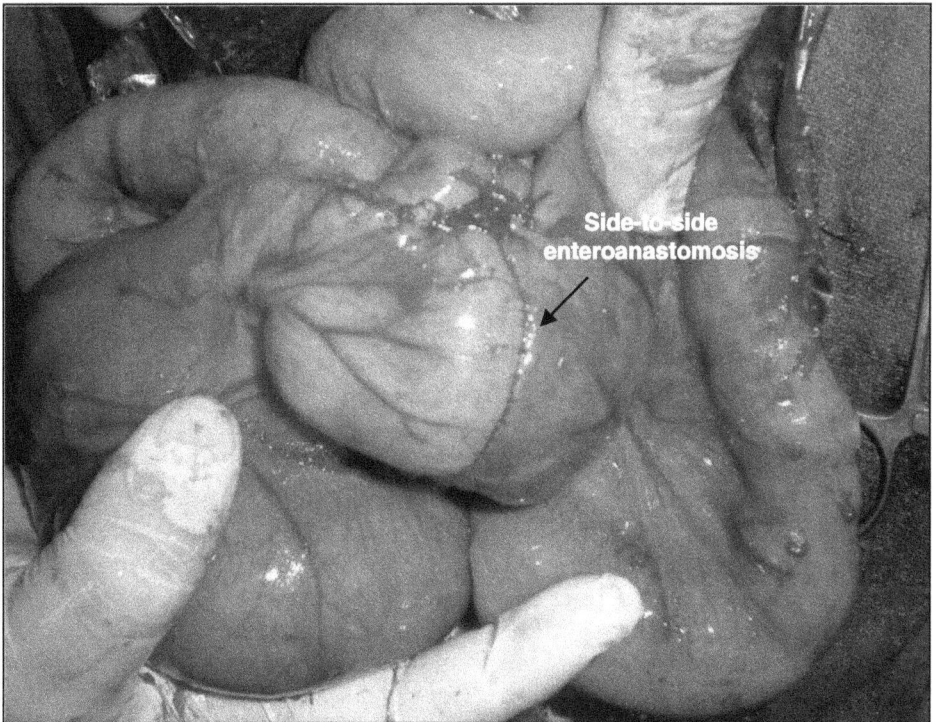

Figure 13.10: Intussusception Bypass.

Routine post-operative care is given. No intra-operative complication is generally seen.

14

Ventral Herniorrhaphy

A.K. Sharma

Ventral or lateral abdominal hernia is a term used to describe a hernia through any part of the abdominal wall other than a natural orifice. If the hernia is ventral to the stifle skin fold, it is termed as ventral hernia and the rest, e.g, in the flank region, are known as lateral abdominal hernias. Such type of hernias are common in ruminants and are generally acquired in nature.

Any trauma such as a kick in the camel, horn thrust in cattle or violent contact with blunt objects or an abscess in the abdominal cavity may lead to weakening of the abdominal wall subcutaneously. Abdominal distension due to pregnancy or violent straining during parturition may lead to ventral hernia, especially in sheep. An excessively long caudal flank incision for caesarean section in the camel may subsequently cause hernia.

Ventral or lateral hernia is commonly seen along the costal arch, high or low in flank, between the last few ribs or in the ventral abdominal wall near the midline. Size of the hernial opening varies in diameter. It is difficult to palpate the ventral hernial ring during initial stages due to oedema or haematoma in the surrounding tissues. Therefore, it is necessary to wait for the inflammatory swelling to subside before examination is done to confirm the diagnosis. This delay may also facilitate repair as recently traumatized tissues do not hold suture firmly. The hernial sac, formed by the skin and subcutaneous tissues, may or not be lined with the peritoneum. Lack of a peritoneal covering favours the development of adhesions between the viscera and sac, and finally cause incarceration or strangulation. The nature of hernial contents depends on the site of the herniation. A hernia in the left

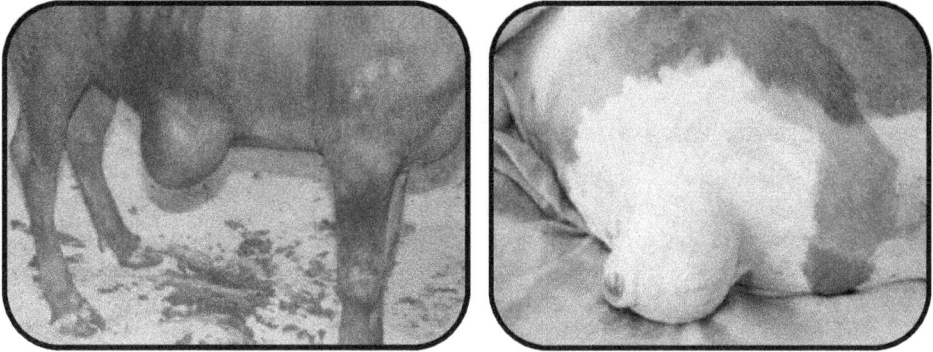

Figure 14.1: Ventral/Umbilical Hernia in Calves.

flank may contain the rumen. In most cases, the condition is harmless and constitutes an unsightly blemish, which is prone to traumatic injuries.

Treatment

The principles of surgical correction of hernia include:

☆ Return of viable contents to their normal position in the abdomen

☆ Secure closure of the neck of hernia, preventing recurrence

☆ Obliteration of the redundant tissue in the sac

☆ Use of patients own tissue wherever possible

When the hernia is apparently harmless, herniorrhaphy is elective and not an emergency operation. It is advisable to delay the surgical repair for at least a week after injury as has already been discussed. However, prolonged delay may cause complications due to loss of muscle elasticity and adhesions sue. If the hernia is complicated due to incarceration or strangulation, immediate surgical intervention is required.

After a linear incision, the skin is freed from all around the swelling. The sac is separated from the ring by blunt dissection and incised. The viscera is freed of any adhesion and returned into the abdominal cavity. The thick mass of fibrous tissue involving the hernial swelling may be resected at the level of the ring and discarded. The edges of the ring are trimmed to provide a raw surface for healing.

The rent in the abdominal wall is then closed by overlapping the edges with a heavy suture material using the technique similar for umbilical hernia. Interrupted sutures can be placed between the overlapping sutures for reinforcement. Excess skin of the sac is removed, and the subcutaneous tissue and skin are apposed with simple continuous and horizontal mattress sutures, respectively. Far-near-near-far tension sutures of 2 No. polydioxanone are used to appose body wall defects. A sterile drainage tube may be placed subcutaneously to prevent accumulation of fluids.

Extensive ventral or lateral hernia may require hernioplasty. Nylon mesh anchored over the defect has proved satisfactory. If a large part of the rumen gets herniated in the flank region, surgery may not be feasible.

Post-operative Management

The amount of feed should be reduced to half for about a week after surgery. A supportive bandage may be placed around the abdomen to relieve tension on the healing tissues. The suture line is treated on general principles of wound care.

Complications are infrequent if the surgery is performed with judicious attention.

☆ *Haematoma*: Due to inadequate haemostasis intraoperatively

☆ *Seroma*: Due to inadequate obliteration of subcutaneous dead space

☆ If the above problem occurs, adopt "Wait and See" approach. Otherwise benign seromas or haematomas may easily get converted to abscesses

☆ Umbilical herniorrhaphy is a straightforward procedure with an excellent prognosis for life and function at any level of activity.

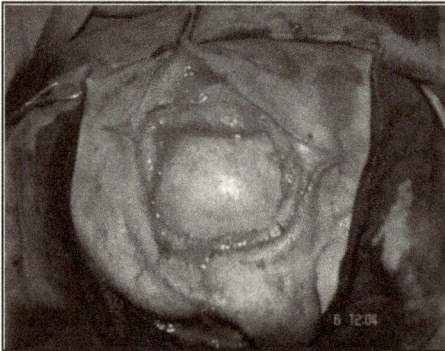

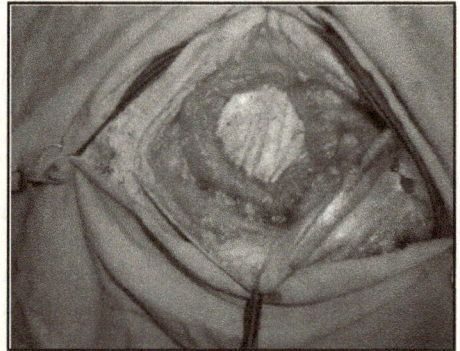

Figure 14.2: Repair of Large Hernias using Biomaterials.

Open Reduction of Hernia

With the availability of safe anaesthetic techniques and improved suture materials, there is little indication for employing a method which is less than certain to correct the hernia. An elliptical incision extending 2 cm beyond the margin of hernial ring cranially and caudally is given. Sutures are inserted 1-2 cm from the edge of the ring and are carried through the full thickness of abdominal wall. Mesh is best placed in an extra-peritoneal position between the internal rectus abdominus muscle sheath and peritoneum. This has greater mechanical advantage than if placed over the defect. Procedure is facilitated by preplacing all the sutures in the mesh.

15

Atresia Ani and Rectovaginal Fistula

Prakash Kinjavdekar

ATRESIA ANI

Atresia is a term that describes a body orifice that is abnormally small or completely closed. Intestinal atresia is a very serious disorder and it is the most common abdominal disease in calves less than 8 days old. Calves born with a form of intestinal atresia can appear normal at birth, but they develop signs 24-48 hours later and most often die within hours of birth if the problem is not surgically corrected.

Atresia ani is defined as the presence of a very small opening or no opening at all at the anus due to a failure of the anal membrane to break down. It is a congenital abnormality, manifested clinically by an absence of faeces, dullness, anorexia with abdominal distension, discomfort and straining at an attempt to defaecate. Atresia coli is a similar condition, where a segment of colon is missing. Both these conditions can be present either alone or in combination with other congenital disorders like rectovaginal fistula.

Etiology

Both atresia ani and atresia coli are congenital defects, which arise due to insult during foetal development and it is thought that atresia ani is an inheritable defect in cattle. There are reports of breed predilection related to the incidence of this condition and Holstein-Friesian calves are at a greater risk than other breeds.

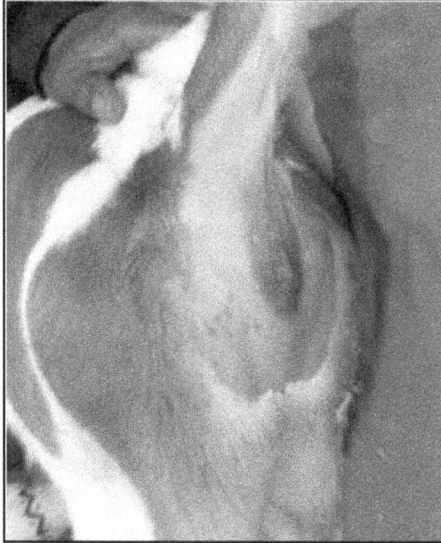

Figure 15.1: A Calf with Atresia Ani.

Another possible etiological factor includes damage to the amniotic vesicle during early pregnancy palpation leading to damage to the blood supply to the foetal intestine.

Symptoms

Calves with atresia ani can show severe signs within hours of birth, while symptoms of atresia coli usually do not appear until 24-48 hours after birth. The affected calf will be unable to pass any faeces so it takes some time for faeces to build up and cause clinical signs. Typical signs of intestinal atresia include decreased appetite, progressive bilateral abdominal distension, the absence of faeces, episodes of straining to defaecate, and occasionally blood-tinged mucous can be found around the rectum. The most characteristic clinical sign is bulging of rectal lumen usually subcutaneously at the normal site of the anus when the abdomen is compressed.

Diagnosis

Lateral abdominal radiograph in calves affected with atresia ani will show a distended, faeces-filled colon with an abrupt end at the level of the rectum. However, abdominal radiographs of calves with atresia coli will show enlarged loops of bowel and absence of faeces in the rectum. Sometimes, giving a barium enema prior to radiography of the abdomen can help determine the level of the defect in cases of atresia coli. Animals with atresia ani are usually easier to diagnose since they will show signs early on and sometimes the imperforate membrane can be palpated.

Surgical Treatment

Treating atresia ani and atresia coli involves surgically opening the blocked orifice. The defect in atresia coli is usually at the level of the spiral loop of the

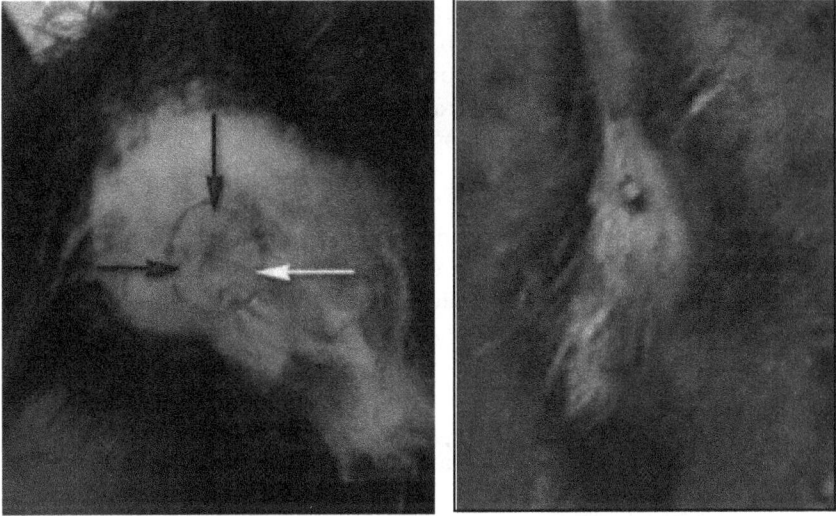

Figures 15.2 and 15.3: Incision for Correction of Atresia Ani; After Correction.

ascending colon, so correction involves removing the defective section of the bowel and reattaching the normal sections. Unfortunately, surgical correction of atresia coli has a poor overall success rate, with a short-term survival rate of less than 50 per cent and a long-term survival rate of less than 35 per cent.

For surgical correction, 2-3 ml of 1 per cent lignocaine solution is injected epidurally, and the animal is restrained in sternal recumbency with the hind feet pulled in a slightly cranial direction. After routine aseptic preparation of the surgical site, a 1-2 cm diameter circular incision is made through the skin and subcutaneous tissue at the site where the anus would normally be located. The skin edges are retracted with Allis forceps held by an assistant. A distended blind-ended rectum is easily located by digital exploration in pelvic midline. Careful blunt dissection in a cranial direction is carried out, followed by gentle pulling of the rectal pouch with a pair of tissue forceps (rectal pull-through procedure) in a caudal direction. If this does not allow the rectum to be identied, it may be grasped via left ank exploratory celiotomy and moved in a caudal direction by simultaneous traction through the pelvic canal and manipulation in the abdomen. The rectum is sutured to the subcutaneous tissue with four interrupted sutures placed dorsally, ventrally and bilaterally into the rectum to maintain it in position and then rectal pouch is incised vertically for 1-2 cm length, which will lead to spurting of meconium from the lumen. The extra-rectal meconium should be removed with damp swabs, but the wound should not be irrigated as it could push infection cranially. Maintaining a lumen of minimum 2 cm diameter may require frequent dilatation of the opening for several weeks because surgical wound healing results in localized necrosis.

Intraoperatively, the presence of anal sphincter muscles is rarely evident. Faecal incontinence is therefore a frequent complication of surgical correction of atresia ani. A single stab incision through the perineum into the rectum is not successful, as stricture and obstruction are likely to occur. If there is a sizable portion of rectum (and descending colon) missing, surgery is exceedingly difficult because the short mesocolon does not readily stretch, and in such cases, surgery should be discouraged. Before suturing the rectum to the perineal skin, any rectovaginal or urethral fistula needs to be located and transected in the female. This is usually done easily by exploring the vaginal opening and fistula with a blunt instrument.

Post-operative Care

Broad spectrum antibiotic is administered for 3-5 days to prevent surgical wound infection. Topical application of povidone iodine solution as well as fly repellant cream around the wound region is advised. Dilatation of the anal opening by frequently inserting a finger to prevent any stricture formation due to wound contraction is also advised.

Prevention

Preventing intestinal atresia in cattle cannot be fully accomplished because the causes of this abnormality are not fully understood. However, there are measures to take to reduce the incidence in a herd. Given the Holsteins have an increased incidence of atresia coli, it is evident that it may be an autosomal recessive trait in the breed. Hence, it is advisable to cull any affected calves and not attempt surgical correction of atresia coli. Additionally, the possibility that damage of blood supply to the developing faetal intestine during the first 6 weeks of pregnancy can cause atresia coli, warrants gentle palpation techniques during this sensitive period of gestation.

RECTOVAGINAL FISTULA

Rectovaginal fistula is a fistulous tract that connects the vagina and rectum. It has been reported to occur in many species but the condition is more common in mares than in most domestic animals. During parturition, the front foot of foal/calf, in an anterior dorsosacral presentation, typically perforates the dorsal aspect of the vestibule and enters the rectum. The foot is withdrawn and leaves a defect between the rectum and vagina. It can also occur at parturition when the annular fold of the hymen at the vaginovestibular junction obstructs passage of the foal's forefoot or nose. Rectovaginal fistula has been also reported to be seen usually in conjunction with imperforate anus (atresia ani) in neonatal animals.

Although minor laceration to the perineum does not require surgery, major ones will affect reproductive performance and require surgical correction. Unlike some other species, the constrictor vestibuli muscle and cervix of the cow help prevent infection, which allows some cattle with complete perineal lacerations to become pregnant.

Etiology

Most of the rectovaginal injuries occur at the time of foaling, either as a result of an oversized or malpositioned foetus, or because of excessive manipulation during assisted delivery. Rectovaginal fistula can also be encountered as a complication arising due to failure of third-degree perineal laceration repair. Severe

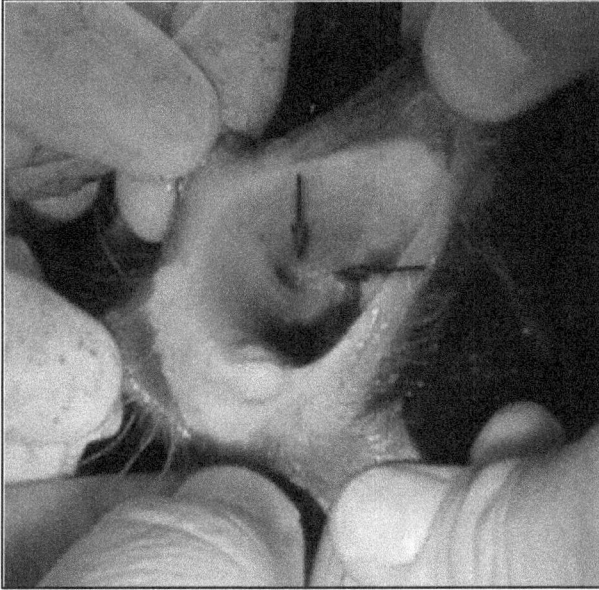

Figure 15.4: Rectovaginal Fistula in a Calf.

trauma that leaves a wide opening between the rectum and vagina has also been reported, but are rarely encountered in clinical practice.

Diagnosis

In newborn animals, there may be clinical signs of passage of faeces through the vulva, and sometimes the owner complaints that faeces and urine are coming through a common vaginal opening. Diagnosis may be confirmed by barium enema, which outlines the extension of the defect into the vagina.

In cases with history of recent assisted foaling in mares, there are increased chances of getting this condition. Faecal contamination of the reproductive tract commonly results in vaginitis and endometritis, and loss of the constrictor vulva muscle or functional rectal sphincter, or both, leading to pneumovagina/wind sucker condition.

Surgical Management

Identification of the fistula, surgical correction and reestablishment of the normal anatomic structures are imperative. The surgical management has two parts, immediate treatment and delayed surgical repair. Repair in the acute stage should be avoided as far as possible because the tissue is very oedematous and contaminated with faeces, and some tissues may not be viable. Repair can be delayed for 4-6 weeks to allow healing of the injured tissues because the defect size can be reduced markedly as a result of wound contraction. Some smaller defects have been reported to heal completely. Initial therapy should include daily wound care and cleaning of the contaminated tissues.

For surgical repair, animal is restrained in standing stocks, the rectum is evacuated of faeces, and the tail is retracted to one side. Some surgeons like to construct a rectal tampon from an orthopaedic stockinette filled with cotton and secured at the ends with umbilical tape. After the administration of lignocine epidurally, the rectum is evacuated and the perineum prepared for aseptic surgery. Perioperative antimicrobials are indicated. A transverse incision is made between the rectum and vagina. By using a combination of sharp and blunt dissection in a horizontal plane, the fistula is exposed. Ideally 2/3 of the thickness of the shelf should be with the rectum and 1/3 with the vaginal shelf. Dissection is continued 3-4 cm rostral to the fistula. The rectal defect is closed transversely (because the musculature of the rectum is primarily circular and sutures placed perpendicular to the muscle fibers are subject to less stress than the sutures placed parallel to the direction of the muscle fibers) by using No. 0/1 absorbable sutures in a simple interrupted pattern placed in the sub-mucosa, with care taken not to penetrate the rectal mucosa. Successful repairs have also been reported with longitudinal closure of the rectum. Either technique is adequate if there is good tissue apposition with little tension. The vaginal defect is closed in next step. Many surgeons advocate a continuous horizontal mattress pattern in a longitudinal direction (because its muscle fibers are primarily longitudinal) so that the two suture rows (rectal and vaginal suture layer) are at right angles to each other and the vaginal mucosa is everted. The incised skin of the perineal body is closed with interrupted non-absorbable monofilament sutures, which are removed 10-14 days later.

Post-operative Care

Post-operative treatment of the mare after repair of a rectovaginal fistula usually includes administration of broad-spectrum antimicrobial drugs (Procaine penicillin G (20,000 IU/kg, IM, BID) and non-steroidal anti-inflammatory drugs like flunixin meglumine (1 mg/kg, IV, BID) for 7 days. The mare should receive tetanus prophylaxis, if she has not received it previously. Post-operatively, temporary atony of the rectum, pain, or solid faeces can cause constipation and increased exertion for defaecation may cause dehiscence. To prevent this, it is important to manage the diet, administer analgesic therapy and if needed careful manual evacuation of the rectum. Hence, faeces should be kept soft and scanty for at least 10 days by modification of the diet and administration of a faecal softener (mineral oil or raw linseed oil). Repair can usually be safely evaluated on the 9th or 10th post-operative day. Defects in the repair are best detected with palpation of tissue between a hand inserted into the rectum and a hand inserted into the vestibule. Mares that strain excessively after surgery should receive epidural anlgesia and sedation, and the cause of straining should be eliminated. Causes of straining include faecal impaction of the rectum and bacterial cystitis. Mares that are reproductively healthy before development of a rectovaginal laceration or fistula are usually able to eliminate bacteria from the tubular genital tract within one estrous cycle. In mares that still have a functional vestibulovaginal seal after a rectovestibular laceration or fistula, endometritis may not develop, provided the tear is caudal to the seal. Those mares that have developed endometritis appear to be capable of rapidly resolving inflammation after perineal repair. Natural breeding should not be allowed for at least 3 months after the repair of a third-degree perineal laceration.

Prognosis is usually guarded. Complications are common and include faecal and urinary incontinence. Faecal incontinence arises due to rectal stricture during healing period, while urinary incontinence arises because of ascending infection leading to cystitis. Other complications include suture dehiscence and recurrence of the condition.

Prevention

Care and attention during difficult deliveries to reposition the foal or prevent a foot from penetrating the septum may be possible. Make sure that anyone doing a rectal examination is well-qualified and that the mare is properly sedated or restrained.

16

Perineal Laceration and Rectal Affections

Kiranjeet Singh and Aswathy Gopinathan

PERINEAL LACERATION

Third degree perineal lacerations in equines are most severe form of perineal injury and involve all layers of vestibule, perineal body and rectum, with disruption of the anus. Severe anterior tears that penetrate the peritoneal cavity can lead to rapid death as a result of massive peritoneal contamination. Those cases which are presented within 4 hours of trauma can successfully be treated by emergency reparative surgery. Treatment at late stage (more than 4-6 hours) is invariably ineffective, as partial breakdown mostly occurs. In such cases healing and granulation of the torn area usually takes 4-6 weeks and hence the surgery is usually delayed till inflammation subsides completely.

Indications

Dystocia, traumatic bleeding or conversion of recto-vaginal fistula into third degree perineal laceration for subsequent repair.

Equipments

Long handled instruments and monofilament absorbable suture materials are required. Self-retaining retractors (Balfour, modified Finichietto) and a good light source (floor lamps, head lamps or fibre-optic lights) are useful.

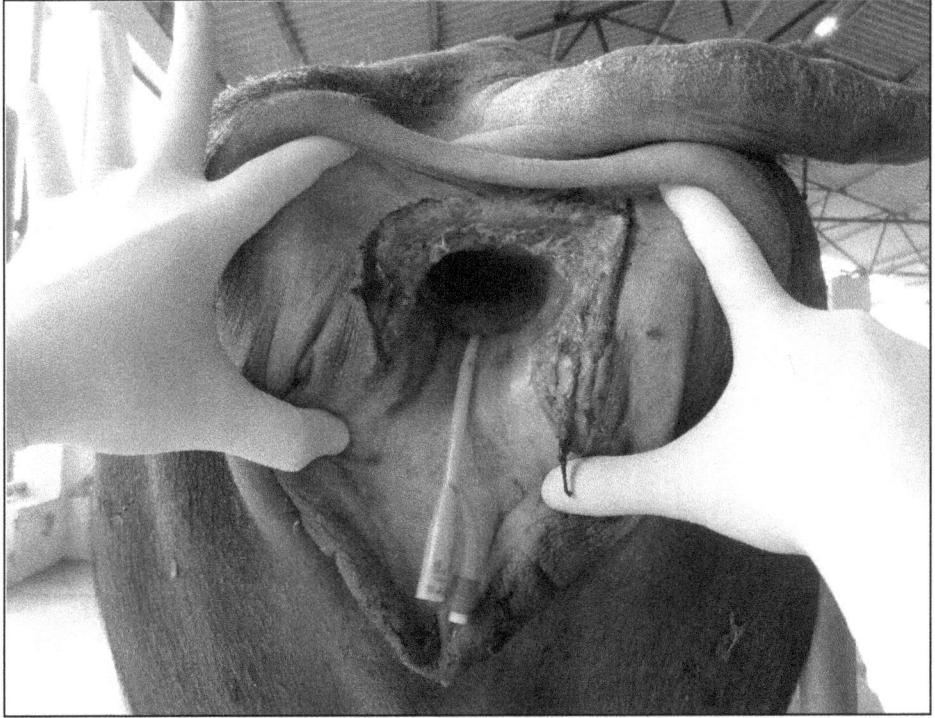

Figure 16.1: Photograph of the Buffalo with Second Degree Perineal Laceration before Surgery.

Preparation and Positioning

Surgery is delayed for 4-6 weeks following laceration to allow wound contraction and inflammation to subside. Delaying surgery allows the wound edges to strengthen and become clearly defined before repair is attempted. A gruel or pasture diet is fed 3-5 days prior to surgery, and the mare is fasted 1 day before the surgery. The mare is restrained standing in a stock and surgery is performed under epidural analgesia with or without sedation. Surgery can also be performed in a patient induced with general anaesthesia in lateral recumbency. After induction of anaesthesia, the tail is secured and retracted. Faecal material is removed from the rectum and vagina. The perineal region is rinsed followed by cleansing of rectal and vaginal lumens with a dilute povidone-iodine solution. The perineal region is aseptically prepared.

Procedure

One- or two- staged technique can be applied, former is preferred but latter should be performed when there is excessive tension at the suture line. No distinct advantage or disadvantage exists between these techniques. Principles for all techniques include initial creation of rectal and vaginal shelves, minimal tissue tension and maintaining a soft faecal consistency after surgery.

**Figure 16.2–16.4: Photograph of a Mare with
Third Degree Perineal Laceration Before Surgery.**

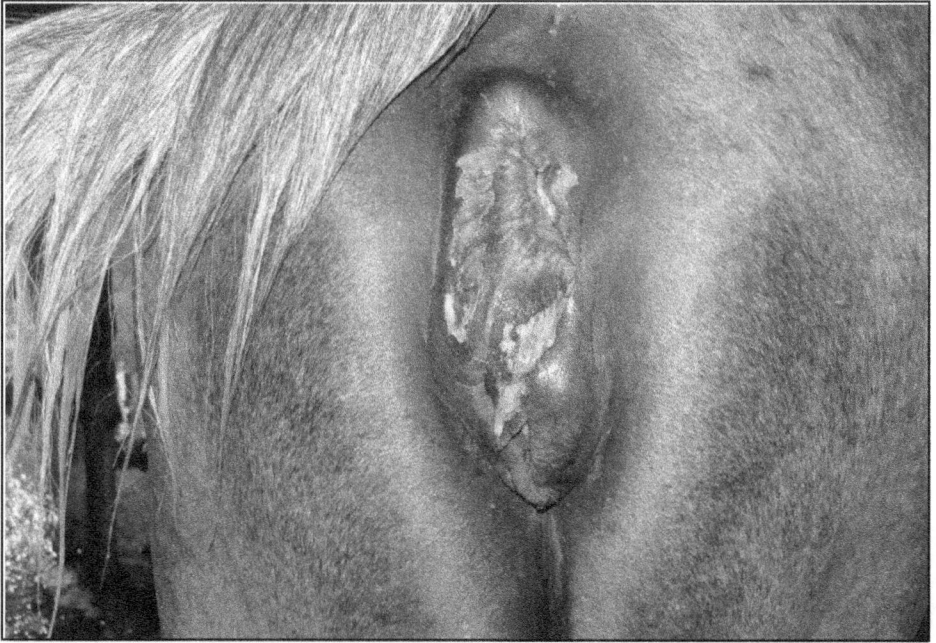

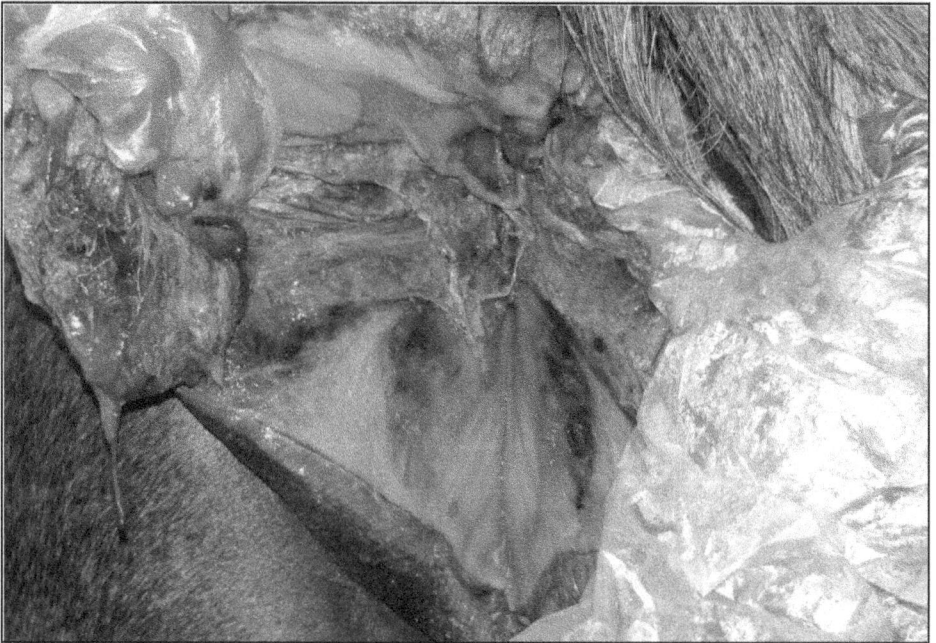

Contd...

Figure 16.2–16.4–*Contd...*

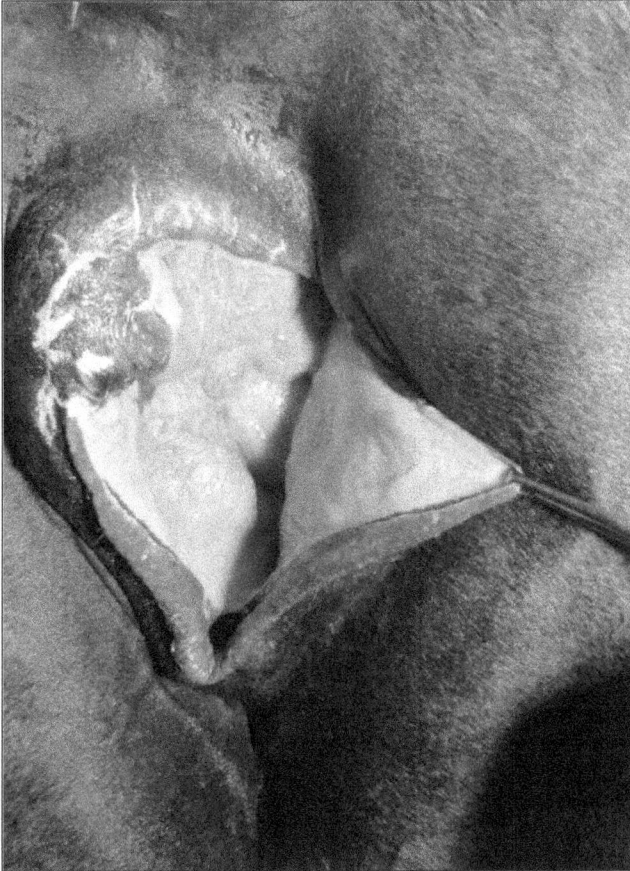

Towel clamps or retention sutures are positioned along the dorso-lateral and ventro-lateral aspects of the defect to provide exposure. The cranial extent of laceration is extended 3 cm, creating a rectal and vaginal shelf. Dissection is continued laterally and caudally along the scar tissue line into the submucosa until the tissue flaps created can be apposed on midline without tension. Both mucosal surfaces are dissected 2 cm or more.

One Stage Repair (Goetz Technique)

Using No. 1 absorbable suture, a six bite pattern is used to close the recto-vaginal shelf. The suture pattern should begin within the vaginal lumen, allowing the knot to be secured within the vaginal lumen. Sutures are positioned approximately 1 cm apart, the suture pattern includes the vaginal mucosa but does not penetrate the rectal mucosa. The vaginal mucosa is closed over the newly created recto-vaginal shelf with No. 0 absorbable suture using a continuous horizontal mattress pattern. The rectal mucosa is left to heal by second intention. Closure of

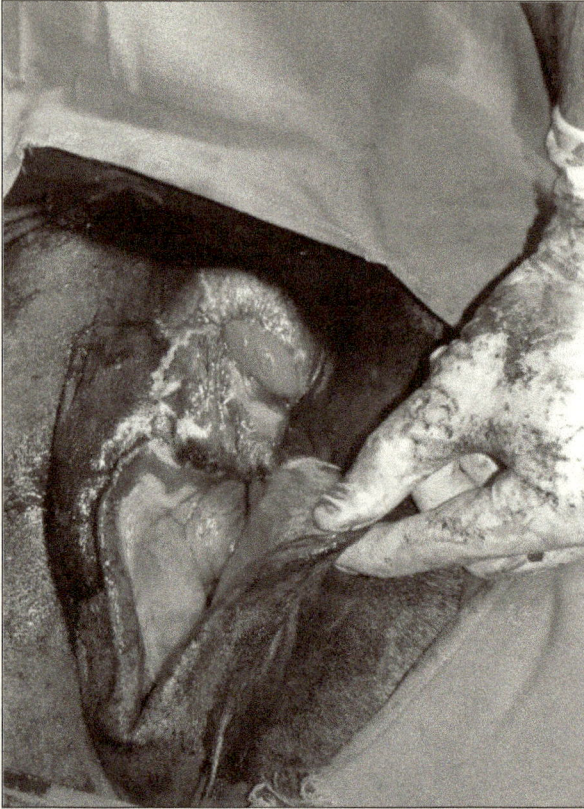

Figure 16.5: Photograph of a Mare After First Stage Repair of Third Degree Perineal Laceration.

the recto-vaginal shelf and vaginal mucosa should extend to the cutaneous perineum. Caslick's procedure is then performed to appose the vulvar opening.

Two Stage Repair (Aanes Technique)

The vaginal mucosa is inverted into the vaginal lumen with No. 0 absorbable suture material using Cushing or Lambert pattern. This suture pattern is continued caudally to reconstruct the cranial half of the defect and then tied but not cut. Using No. 1 absorbable suture, purse string sutures are made to close the recto-vaginal shelf. Sutures are positioned approximately 1 cm apart and should not pass through the vaginal or rectal mucosa. If an excessive amount of tension or dead space is present, partial tightening of the purse-string sutures along with saggitally oriented simple interrupted sutures will help obliterate dead space. Once the cranial half of the recto-vaginal shelf is reconstructed, closure of the vaginal mucosa is completed, followed by closure of the remaining caudal half of the recto-vaginal shelf. Optionally, the rectal mucosa may be inverted into the rectal lumen with No. 2-0 absorbable suture material using Cushing or Lambert pattern. Closure of the recto-vaginal shelf is continued to the level of the cutaneous perineum.

Closure of the perineal body is performed 3-4 weeks after the first surgery if recto-vestibular shelf is completely healed. If dehiscence occurs or a fistula is present, the first stage should be repeated. Closure of the perineal body is performed using perineal body reconstruction technique. A triangular section of the vestibular mucosa is reflected ventrally and removed from each side, with a triangle apex pointing cranially and the base along the mucocutaneous junction of the perineum. Closure of the ventral vestibular mucosal margins should be performed in a cranial to caudal manner with No. 2-0 absorbable suture in a simple continuous pattern. Deep perineal tissues should be apposed with No. 2-0 absorbable sutures using a simple interrupted pattern. Perineal skin is apposed with No. 0 non absorbable sutures using Ford interlocking pattern.

Recently a new modification of the surgical technique has been applied and it showed healing by first intention, and subjects had good post-surgical fertility. In this technique, the rectovestibular shelf was corrected with three parallel 'circular' continuous suture rows distributed along the longitudinal axis of the vagina, and the perineal body was reconstructed with three divergent simple continuous rows.

Post-operative Care

☆ Exercise restriction

☆ Medications: Tetanus prophylaxis, broad-spectrum antibiotic are administered for 7-10 days; NSAIDs for 3-5 days

☆ Suture removal: Perineal and Caslick's sutures should be removed 10-14 days after surgery

☆ Dietary modification: Free choice access to grass, a gruel diet or both should be provided for 30 days with gradual return to normal diet. Occasionally mineral oil should be added to maintain soft faecal consistency

☆ Others: Sexual rest is recommended until the following breeding season.

Expected Outcome

Primary healing is reported to occur in approximately 70-90 per cent of repaired third degree perineal laceration cases. Short term complications such as dehiscence or fistula formation are reported to occur in 12-24 per cent of all surgical repairs (2, 4, 6, and 7). Third degree perineal lacerations recur in 5-50 per cent of the foaling mares due to the inelasticity of the resultant scar tissue.

Complications

Suture dehiscence and subsequent fistula development are possible. These complications can be avoided with precise dissection, adequate tissue purchases and reduced tension on apposed tissues. Fistula formation may result in failure to conceive due to endometritis, pneumovagina if continued faecal contamination of the vaginal lumen. Uro-vagina may be a consequence of the mare's natural perineal conformation or the result of altering the perineal conformation during the recto-vaginal fistula repair and can be addressed with an urethroplasty procedure. Mares should be monitored during subsequent foaling because the fibrous tissue from the repair may reduce the elasticity of the birth canal and predispose the mare to additional birthing trauma. As the sutures are progressively placed in the caudal tissue, care must be taken to avoid the narrowing of the rectal lumen, which will predispose the mare to tenesmus and constipation.

RECTAL PROLAPSE

Etiology

Prolonged tenesmus or straining due to rectal inflammation and irritation, diarrhoea, enteritis or parasites, and during act of parturition. Intestinal neoplasia, foreign bodies, perineal hernia, constipation and congenital defects. In incomplete prolapse, only mucosa is prolapsed and in complete prolapse, whole thickness rectal wall is involved. Prolapsed mass is more prone to ischaemia and oedema, contamination and trauma.

Diagnosis

Protrusion of mass through anus. Many a times it is associated with vaginal prolapse. Differential diagnosis: Intussusception with prolapse, especially in young dogs, and tumours like venereal granuloma.

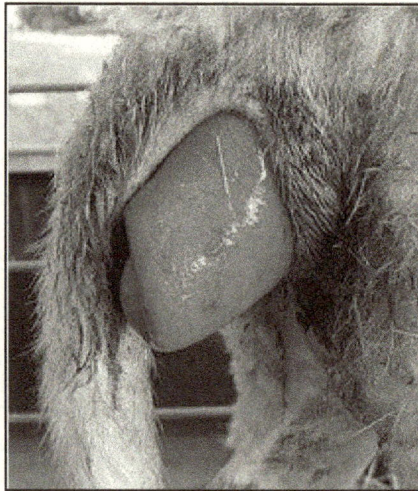

Figure 16.6: Rectal Prolapse in a Buffalo Calf.

Treatment

Fresh Cases

☆ Easy to repose

☆ Lavage with astringent solutions and apply antiseptic ointment + lignocaine jelly before repositioning

☆ Apply purse string suture for 2-3 days, when no signs of straining

☆ Epidural analgesia

☆ Laxative diet for few days

Recurrent/Chronic Prolapse

When severe necrosis, damage of the rectal tissue

☆ Amputation of rectum under epidural analgesia

☆ Comlications include peritonitis from wound dehiscence, stenosis or stricture

RECTAL (SUPRA) ABSCESS

More common in horses but also reported in bovines occupying the perineal tissue, wall or floor of rectum.

Etiology

Trauma and infection or associated with strangles.

Symptoms

Swelling or mass pressing the rectal lumen resulting in colic or scanty/no faeces etc.

Diagnosis

Needle aspiration and cytological examination, and ultrasonography.

Prognosis

If abscess is located anteriorly or ventrally, it may rupture causing peritonitis. Abscessses in the lateral or dorsal wall of rectum or towards the anus generally have good prognosis.

Treatment

Incision is given to evacuate the contents. General principles of abscess management are followed. A tube or catheter is placed to maintain the patency of the incision over abscess. Antibiotic based on culture sensitivity test and anti-inflammatory drugs should be administered. Laxatives are advised along with less diet for few days.

17

Management of Urolithiasis in Ruminants

T.B. Sivanarayanan and Amarpal

Urolithiasis is one of the oldest documented miseries of the mankind. The condition has been reported from all corners of the world and in all the species of animals. Since the disease is multifactorial in origin, its incidence varies from place to place and time to time. Etiopathogenesis is obscure, identification of the types of calculi is not always easy, management is difficult and frustrating, especially in ruminants, both for veterinarians and animal owners. The disease thus causes heavy mortality and consequently economic losses to the marginal and poor farmers. Blockage of urethra leading to obstruction to urine flow is the clinical situation demanding immediate surgical intervention. Urethral obstruction, if not relieved in time, leads to rupture of urinary bladder and subsequently diffused, acute, severe fibrinous peritonitis. The abrupt release of large quantities of urine in the abdomen may lead to cardiovascular disturbances resulting in death of the animal. Therefore, it is always advisable to initiate the treatment as early as possible. Approaches to surgical management have changed in the recent past, and simpler and better techniques have been developed, which have reduced the mortality to a great extent in cases suffering from urolithiasis. Some of the useful surgical techniques are described in the following text.

Surgical Managements of Urolithiaisis in Goats and Calves

Urethral Process Amputation

Urethral process is reported as the most common site of calculi lodgment in goats. Urethral process amputation has, therefore, been the most common surgical technique used as first line of treatment of obstructive urolithiasis. Though reports on extrusion of glans penis without preputiotomy are available, it may be difficult to extrude glans penis in immature small ruminants owing to normal attachment of glans penis to prepuce. The procedure is performed under local or lumbosacral epidural analgesia induced with 2 per cent lignocaine. The animal is restrained in right lateral recumbency with left hind limb pulled backward. Ventral abdomen from umbilicus to anterior border of scrotum is prepared for aseptic surgery by shaving, proper scrubbing and painting with povidone-iodine solution. Glans penis is palpated at the tip of penis and ventral midline skin incision of 2 cm is given over the glans. Penis is freed from subcutaneous fascia and gently pulled out. An incision is made in the prepuce to expose the glans. Urethral process is freed from adjacent tissue. A small incision is made in the urethral process at its base and a poly vinyl chloride (PVC) catheter of appropriate size is passed into the urethra as far caudally as possible. Urethral process is then resected from its base. The other end of catheter is passed cranially so as it cames out through preputial orifice. Preputiotomy incision is closed by simple continuous pattern using 3/0 PGA or catgut. Skin incision is closed by No. 1 silk suture using horizontal mattress suturing technique.

Urethrotomy

Removal of uroliths by urethrotomy is the first line of treatment in many practices. In goat urethrotomy is usually performed at post-scrotal site as almost entire length of urethra can be examined through this site. The animal is restrained on the operation table in right lateral recumbency under lumbosacral epidural analgesia. The left hind limb is pulled dorsally and cranially, and tied to the table. Post-scrotal region from the level of caudal border of scrotum to the infra-anal area is prepared for aseptic surgery. A 2 cm long skin incision is given on midline about one inch posterior to the scrotum. Penis is exposed by dissecting subcutaneous fascia and muscles, and exteriorised by gentle traction so as to straighten the sigmoid flexure. Penis is palpated for the presence of any calculus in urethra and adequate length of incision is given over the calculus. The calculus is removed through the incision and a sterilize PVC catheter of appropriate size is passed through the incision in urethra first caudally as far as possible and then cranially so that it comes out through the preputial orifice. Urethral incision or rupture is closed by PGA No. 5/0 in single layer of simple continuous suture pattern. Subcutaneous musculature and fascia are closed with catgut No. 3/0. Skin is then closed in horizontal mattress pattern using surgical silk or nylon thread No. 1.

Urethrostomy

Permanent ischial urethrostomy helps in eliminating the most commonly affected segment of urethral tract, and thus prevents the recurrence. The goat is restrained in dorsal or lateral recumbency. Sacrococcygeal or lumbosacral epidural anaesthesia or local infiltration with 2 per cent lignocaine can be administered. The perineal area extending from the anus to the scrotum is clipped and prepared for the surgery. Skin incision of about 4 cm is made about 2 cm proximal to the caudal border of the scrotum. Adequate blunt dissection is necessary to allow the penis to be exteriorized without excessive tension. To avoid placing the urethrostomy in tissues likely damaged by sharp calculi, the site chosen for urethrostomy should lie proximal to the distal bend of the sigmoid flexure. In cases of urethral rupture, it may be advantageous to transect the penis distal to the urethrostomy site; this will facilitate drainage of urine from the tissues of the inguinal region and prevent infection in devitalized tissue. The dorsal penile vessels are ligated imme-diately proximal to the transection site. The penis is transected and the distal segment excised, a horizontal wedge resection of the cavernosum of the stump is performed, and the cavernosum is closed to limit haemorrhage. The penis is then re-positioned so that the stump is located at the distal apex of the skin incision. If the distal penis is not to be excised, the dorsal penile vessels are left intact.

To hold the exteriorized segment of penis in place, a horizontal mattress suture of monofilament, non-absorbable material is placed through the skin and into the tunica albuginea of the penis on each side of the distal apex of the skin incision. Alternatively, the tunica albuginea can be secured with absorbable suture to the subcutis of the apex of the distal incision. The urethra is incised in a vertical length of approximately 3-4 cm. With proper positioning of the penis, the urethral incision should lie immediately adjacent to the skin incision. If the skin incision is judged to be of excessive length, it can be closed to create a skin incision that more closely aligns with the edges of the incised urethra. A 0 to 3-0 monofilament, nonabsorbable suture material is used to appose the edges of the urethral mucosa to the adjacent skin edges, thus creating a spatulated urethral orifice. The dorsal and ventral apices of the urethral incision are sutured to the corresponding apices of the skin incision. A simple interrupted pattern or several small sections of simple continuous pattern are used to complete the suturing of urethral mucosa to the skin. Meticulous apposition of the urethral mucosa to the skin is necessary to limit haemorrhage from the corpus spongiosum, prevent urine leakage into the subcutis, and create a permanent stoma.

Tube Cystostomy

Tube cystostomy is a urinary diversion or urethral bypass technique, in which a Foley's catheter is placed into the urinary bladder lumen via a small skin incision. It has been used in the treatment of urethral obstruction, urethral rupture or ruptured urinary bladder in small ruminants. Urine diversion by Foley's catheter can be done either temporarily in urethral repair/acute urethral obstruction or permanently in bladder cancer or neurogenic bladder atony. Tube cystostomy catheter also provides avenue for normograde contrast cysto-urethrography, which may be beneficial for evaluating the extent of urethral obstruction or urethral integrity post-operatively and therefore, may potentially be used to monitor urethral healing, assess medical therapy for calculi dissolution and determine when the animal should be encouraged to micturate through the urethra by occluding the drainage catheter. The technique can be utilized effectively in the cases of urethral or bladder ruptures in calves and goats. The animal is restrained under lumbosacral epidural analgesia as for cystotomy. Left ventral abdominal area from the level of umbilicus to the scrotum is prepared for aseptic surgery. A 2 cm long paramedian incision is given 5 cm lateral to midline and 2-3 cm cranial to rudimentary teats in prepubic region, so as to facilitate approach to the urinary bladder. A straight artery forceps is passed anteriorly from the incision to a distance of about 15 cm making subcutaneous tunnel, the tip of the artery forceps is brought out of the skin near preputial orifice by making another nick incision. A tract is thus formed for the fixation of Foley's catheter. A No. 14 French Foley's catheter is pulled through the tract with the help of the same artery forceps. Rectus abdominis muscle and its sheath are separated using pointed end scissors. The abdominal viscera are reflected aside, urinary bladder is palpated and is held in position with two fingers. Foley's catheter is anchored to a K-wire by its eye and passed into the urinary bladder (just behind vertex in ventral midline) with a sudden thrust applied to the K-wire without exposing the abdominal organs. As soon as the urine starts coming out from the catheter, the balloon of Foley's catheter is inflated with 5 ml of sterile saline, the K-wire is retracted slowly and then 10 ml of saline is infused into the balloon of the catheter. A purse string suture using a monofilament absorbable suture of 1/0-size is placed in the bladder wall to secure the catheter in place and prevent urine leakage. Care is taken to avoid puncturing of the catheter or its balloon during suture placement. The external end of the catheter is then pulled gently to appose the bladder wall to the body wall at the interior aspect of the incision. The abdominal muscle layer is sutured with No.1 catgut and skin with No.1 silk or nylon. The part of Foley's catheter outside the abdomen is fixed with abdominal wall using 5-6 stay sutures.

Ammonium chloride 500 mg/kg body wt. is given as acidifier to the animals from day 3 of surgery. Urethra is examined for the reestablishment of patency by examining the signs of urination, and if possible by positive contrast cysto-urethrography. Treatment is continued for at least 15 days so as to maintain urine pH within a range of 6.0-6.5. Clamping of Foley's catheter is started from day 5 to encourage urination through prepuce and animal is examined for the signs of urination. Cystotomy catheter is blocked when the urethral passage is clear of

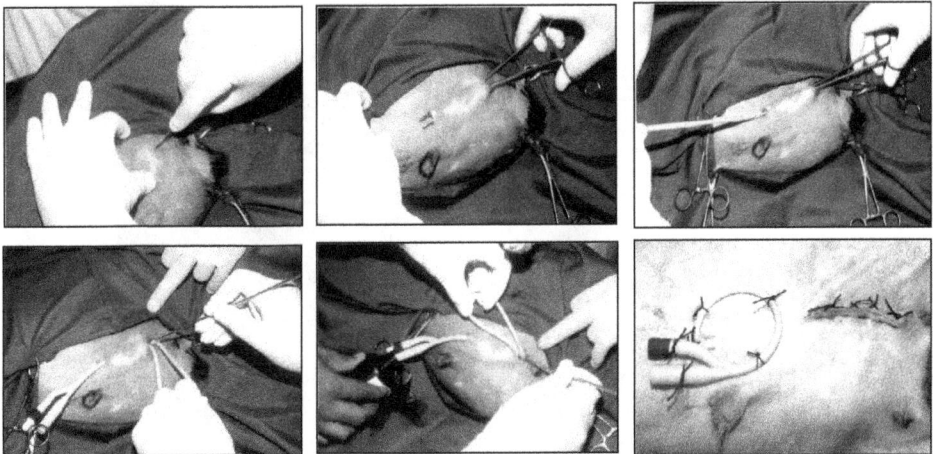

Figure 17.1: Tube Cystostomy in a Goat.

obstruction. Foley's catheter is removed by deflating its balloon and is pulled out of bladder and abdomen 3-4 days after clearance of urethral passage. The tract left by catheter is dressed until healing, which takes place without any complications.

Cystorrhaphy

The most serious sequel to ever increasing pressure of accumulating urine in an untreated case of urethral obstruction is the rupture of urinary bladder. The use of drugs like Frusemide to treat the urethral obstruction in field conditions further aggravates the chances of bladder rupture by increasing the urine production. Repair of the ruptured urinary bladder is the clinical situation requiring cystorrhaphy, whereas cystotomy is indicated to clear the bladder of calculi with and without urohydropropulsion. Lumbosacral epidural anaesthesia is generally adequate, however, infiltration of the abdominal wall with lignocaine is also required at times.

The animal is restrained on the table in right lateral or dorsal recumbency, and the left hind limb is lifted and tied to the far side of the table to expose the caudal ventral abdomen. Left ventral abdominal area from the level of umbilicus to the scrotum is prepared for aseptic surgery. A paramedian skin incision, 2-3 cm lateral to the prepuce, measuring about 10 cm is made. The caudal end of the incision is extended up to the level of the rudimentary teats. The subcutis is incised to expose the external rectus sheath. The incision is continued through the rectus abdominis muscle and the peritoneum is incised to open the abdominal cavity. In cases of rupture of urinary bladder the accumulated urine in abdomen is drained slowly so as to avoid shock. The urinary bladder is located and pulled out through the abdominal incision by gentle traction. Rent in the bladder is identified and closed by continuous Lambert sutures reinforced by Cushing sutures using 3/0 polyglycolic acid. Urinary bladder is examined for any leakage by applying gentle pressure. Abdominal cavity is lavaged with normal saline solution and then closed routinely by suturing muscle and peritoneal layers together with 1/0 chromic catgut by simple continuous pattern. Subcutaneous layer may be sutured with absorbable suture of

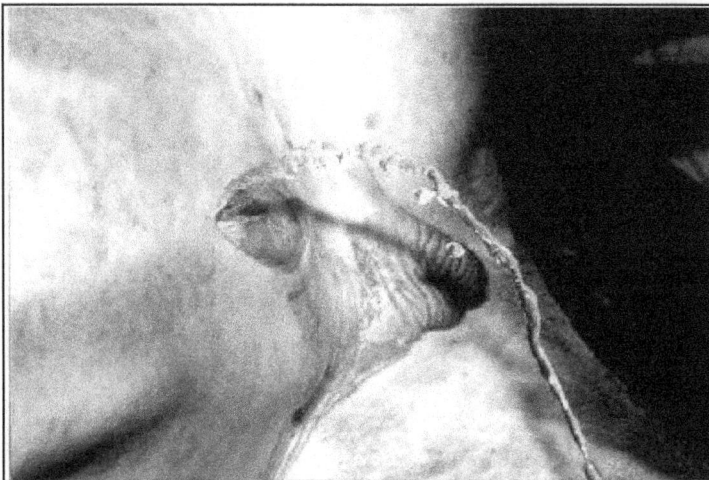

Figure 17.2: Tube Cystostomy after Cystorrhaphy.

2/0 size in continuous pattern. Skin is closed by 1/0 surgical silk or nylon by horizontal mattress sutures.

Surgical Managements of Urolithiasis in Bullocks

The most common site of obstruction in cattle is distal part of sigmoid flexure adjacent to the attachment of the retractor penis muscle, but calculus can get lodged anywhere between the ischial arch and the sigmoid flexure, and in a few cases at the neck of the urinary bladder, or even the tip of urethra.

Obstruction to the flow of urine can lead to futile and painful attempts by the animal to void urine. The clinical signs of retained urine become apparent within 24 hr after complete urethral obstruction, and rupture of the bladder occurs within 72 hr and the animal gets temporary relief. If proper treatment is delayed further, the animal may die in 4-5 days, but some animals may survive longer. Since sigmoid flexure is the most common site, post-scrotal urethrotomy is generally performed for the removal of the calculus, however, when the calculus is lodged at other sites, the urethrotomy incision needs to be made accordingly.

Post-Scrotal Urethrotomy

In cases where the urinary bladder is intact, post-scrotal urethrotomy alone may relieve the obstruction. The animal is restrained in right lateral recumbency and the midline area extending from the scrotum to the infra-anal arch is prepared for surgery. Local anaesthesia is achieved using line infiltration technique; caudal epidural analgesia is discouraged as it may reduce the tonicity of the bladder. A 10-15 cm long midline incision is made extending upward from the caudal border of scrotum. The skin and subcutaneous tissue are incised, the muscles dissected bluntly; haemorrhage is generally minimal in this area. The penis in this area can be felt as a hard cord like structure. A curved artery forceps is passed under the penis and it is levered. A gentle incision may be given over the penis to remove the fascial covering around the penis, while avoiding cutting the penile veins. Sigmoid flexure is straightened and an adequate length of the penis is exteriorized. The urethra lies in the urethral groove on the ventral aspect of the penis. It passes between the insertions of the retractor penis muscle. The urethra is thoroughly examined by holding the penis in palm and palpating the urethra by passing the thumb over it. In bullocks the obstructing calculus can be felt as a hard and irregular bulging in the passage of urethra. A nick incision is given on the urethra at the site of the uroliths which is then pressed out or removed by holding it with the help of a small artery forceps. When the calculus is located above the sigmoid flexure towards the ischial arch, it can be palpated in many cases by passing the index finger along the penis. The incision is extended up to the level of calculus lodgement.

After removing the calculus, a snugly fitting sterilize polyethylene catheter is passed into the urethra, first to the proximal end as far as possible, as many times it is not possible to pass the catheter up to the bladder from this incision. The other end of the catheter is passed from the same incision to distal urethra so that it comes out through the preputial orifice. Flow of urine through the catheter indicates correct placement of the catheter and clearing of the obstruction. The outer end of

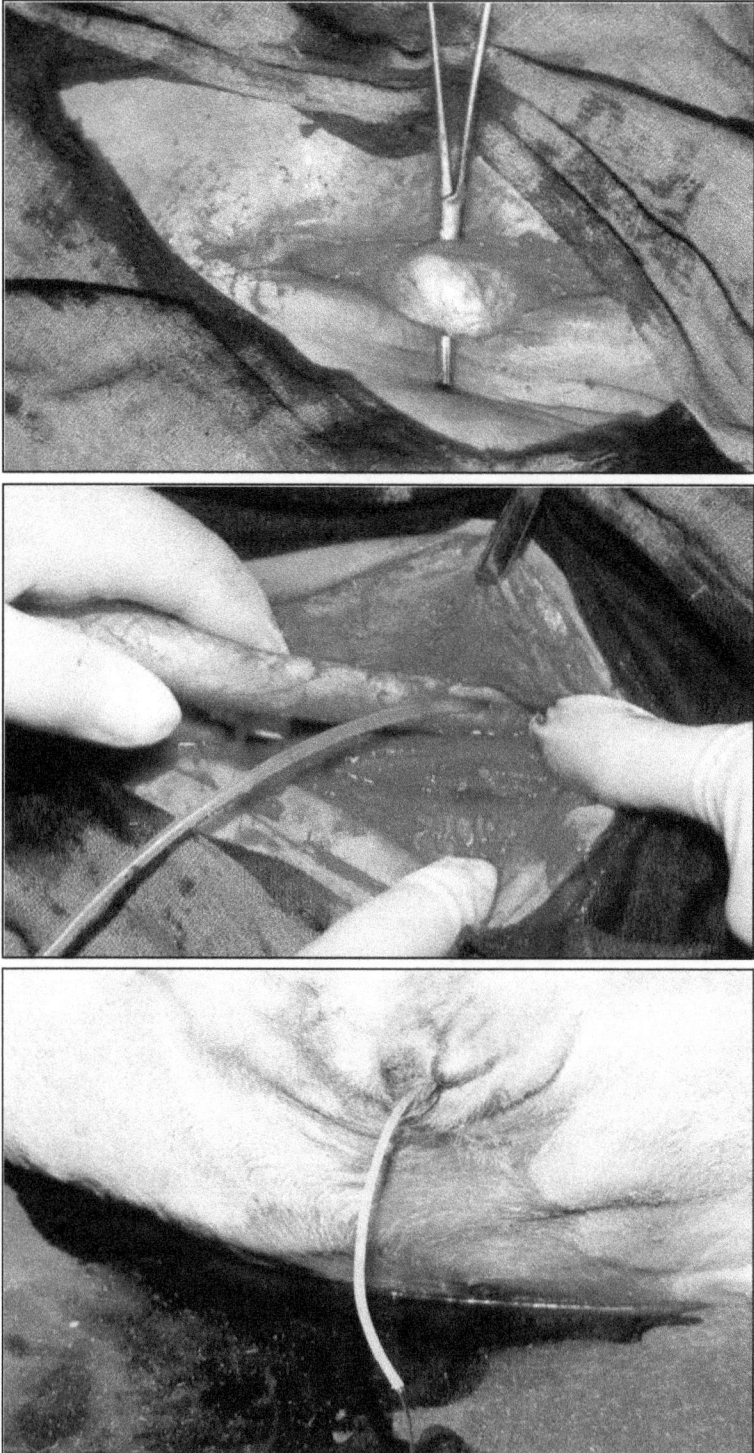

Figure 17.3: Placement of PVC Catheter in Urethra after Removal of Calculi.

the catheter is anchored with the preputial sheath to prevent its dislodgement. Some workers do not advise suturing of urethral wound, because if catheter is snugly fitted and there is no seepage of urine from the urethral wound, it heals automatically. However, it is recommended to suture the urethra by simple continuous pattern using an absorbable suture material. Muscles are not sutured. Subcutaneous tissue is closed with interrupted sutures using absorbable suture material and the skin with mattress sutures using nonabsorbable material like nylon 2-0. The catheter is allowed to stay in the urethra up to 20 days.

Cystorrhaphy

Rupture of the urinary bladder is very common in bullocks after urethral obstruction. Delayed diagnosis of the obstructive urolithiasis and delayed presentation of the case to the clinics frequently result in rupture of the urinary bladder and development of "water belly" condition. It is reported that discrete dorsal tears may sometimes heal spontaneously and ventral tears require surgical intervention; however, once the abdomen is opened to locate the site of obstruction, it is advisable to carry out cystorrhaphy. The repair of the urinary bladder is preferably undertaken after removal of the calculus from the urethra because normograde urethral catheterization can be performed at the time of cystorrhaphy.

Cystorrhaphy can be undertaken through different approaches like para-anal, infra-anal and ventral; however, left paralumbar fossa approach is preferred as it provides sufficient space for manipulation of bladder in standing animal. The surgery can be done under paravertebral or local infiltration analgesia. After achieving local anaesthesia and preparation of the site for surgery, about 20 cm long skin incision is made in the most caudal part of paralumbar fossa. The abdominal fascia, muscles and the peritoneum are incised to enter the abdominal cavity. The laparotomy incision should be large enough to allow the entry of both hands into the abdominal cavity. The urine present in the abdomen will gush out and the urine below the level of incision should be siphoned out as much as possible. The urinary bladder is identified and the tear in the urinary bladder is located and the bladder is examined for the presence of any calculus, concretions or blood clots, which are removed before undertaking the repair. Catheterization of the urethra is attempted with a polyethylene catheter having a sterile stylet. The proximal end of the catheter is fenestrated before attempting catheterization. The catheter is passed inside the bladder through the tear and introduced into the urethra up to the entire length of the urethra. The stylet is then pulled out from the proximal end. The catheter is held from the distal end and pulled slowly so that only 2-3 cm of the catheter remains in the urinary bladder. The distal end of the catheter is anchored to the preputial sheath using a non-absorbable suture.

The tear in the bladder ideally should be repaired by applying inverting sutures but may be repaired by applying continuous sutures using absorbable suture material. A second row of continuous suture is applied to avoid leakage. The abdominal cavity is copiously lavaged with saline to remove the traces of the urine before closing the abdominal incision in a routine manner.

Tube Cystostomy in Bullocks

Tube cystostomy has produced excellent results in the management of urolithiasis in small ruminants and dogs. Urethrotomy can be avoided in many cases with the use of this technique. The original technique through the flank or ventral abdomen can not be applied in large animals due to the smaller length of Foley's catheter. The technique of tube cystostomy is, therefore performed through para-anal approach in bullocks.

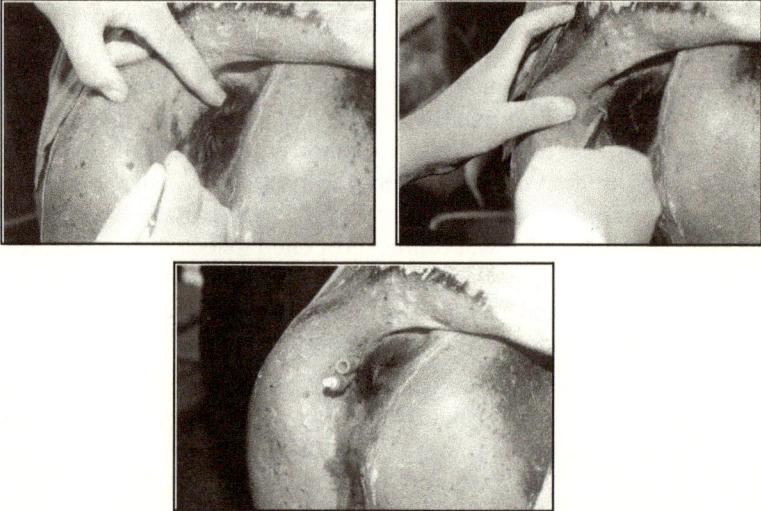

Figure 17.4: Tube Cystostomy in Bullocks through Para-Anal Approach.

A left flank laparotomy is performed in the bullock under paravertebral block and the urine in abdominal cavity is siphoned out. Under caudal epidural analgesia a nick incision is made in perianal fossa lateral to anal opening. An intramedullary pin of 10 mm diameter is used to make a rent in the pelvic diaphragm. A Foley's catheter is then introduced through this tunnel in the pelvic cavity with the help of a 5 mm orthopaedic K-wire. The Foley's catheter is fixed into the bladder on the lateral side near the apex by inserting the hand through the laparotomy incision. The balloon of the catheter is inflated and laparotomy incision closed. The approach is suitable for large animals and can be used to facilitate the healing of urethrotomy incision by providing urinary bypass.

18

Castration of Male Animals

M.R. Fazili

Castration is one of the most frequently performed surgical procedures in veterinary practice. Castration as far back as 7000 BC has been the only early surgery performed in cattle. The common indications of castration are to make the animal docile, for easy management in the presence of female animals, to prevent unwanted animals from breeding, malignant disease or irreparable injury of the testes, to promote weight gain in meat animals, and for correction of scrotal hernia.

Younger animals are generally easier to restrain, have lesser risk of incisional complications and show decreased aggressive behaviour after castration. Bulls castrated prior to puberty grow to a greater height because castration delays closure of the growth plates of their long bones, and the same may be true in other animal species. The preferable ages of castration in cattle (1-2 months), sheep and goats (2-3 weeks) and horse (1-1.5 yrs) have been reported. But in actual practice, the animals may be castrated at any age. Under field conditions, the owner's choice, ease of procedure and intended use of the animal may affect this decision. Whenever possible the extreme climates and the heavy fly seasons should be avoided.

Adequate fasting of the animal preoperatively in all elective surgeries is an important prerequisite for successful outcome. The surgeon should ensure that the correct animal is castrated and obtain a medical history. A brief physical examination to determine the health status is always recommended. The scrotum is examined to confirm the presence of both testes and to determine whether inguinal herniation is present or not. Under field conditions most clinically normal animals can be safely subjected to routine elective surgery without the benefit of laboratory tests. However, the procedure should not be performed on sick animals. The surgeon should wear sterile gloves for all open surgeries and use sterilized instruments. Perioperative antibiotics are also necessary particularly under field conditions.

All techniques of castration in animals have several principles in common: adequate restraint, safety, good anaesthesia, clean surgery, control of haemorrhage, and adequate post-operative drainage. The various popular techniques of castration in male animals could be divided into the following categories:

Ruminants (Cattle, Sheep, Goat)

1) *Closed* (Bloodless techniques):
   a) Emasculatome- Burdizzo
   b) Elastic banding, Elastrator, EZE bander, Calicrate bander
2) *Open techniques*:
   a) Short scrotum method (not sutured)
   b) Newberry knife technique (not sutured)
   c) Unilateral orchiectomy (for unilateral disorders)

Equine and Small Animals

1) *Open Method* – Orchiectomy
   a) Open uncovered or "Open Open" method
   b) Open covered or "Open Closed" method

Quiet stallions those allow palpation of the scrotum and testes with little resentment and without sedation are the best candidates for standing surgery. Typically older calves may be put into a squeeze chute or stocks for bloodless castration. Most of the remaining animal species are castrated in recumbency. Ponies, donkeys, mules and horses with poorly developed testes are also difficult to castrate in standing. Lambs and small goats are held head down, between the operator's knees or head up with the front and hind limbs on each side held together. Calves younger than one month of age are usually restrained in lateral recumbency.

Traditionally analgesics and anaesthetics have not been used for castrating ruminants by closed methods. But several studies conducted in the recent past show increased cortisol level in addition to the typical distress behaviours in animals subjected to castration. Analgesia/anaesthesia should therefore be achieved in all the ruminants of all the ages undergoing castration. Sedation along with local infiltration analgesia (scrotal skin/spermatic cord) should be used in every animal. To avoid local anaesthetic toxicity in small ruminants, the 2 per cent lignocaine hydrochloride should be diluted to 0.5 per cent or 1.0 per cent before use. Xylazine at 0.02-0.1 mg/kg IV or 0.04-0.2 mg/kg IM gives satisfactory sedation. Lower range may be used for goats, debilitated, aged, young or depressed animals. In goats midazolam (0.1-0.2 mg/kg IV) in combination with butorphanol (0.02 mg/kg IV) may be used alternatively. In small animals, several injectable anaesthetic combination protocols (phenothiazine derivatives, benzodiazepines, alpha-2 agonists, opioids, dissociative anaesthetics and ultrashort acting barbiturates) for conducting elective surgeries in dogs have been standardized. Ketamine (5-10 mg/kg) with xylazine (1-2 mg/kg) or diazepam (0.1-0.2 mg/kg) along with atropine (0.02-0.04 mg/kg) premedication is currently the easily available and comparatively economical mixture most frequently used in field settings. For standing castration in equines, sedation with xylazine or a combination of xylazine with butorphanol is recommended. Local anaesthesia is achieved by using an 18-gauge, 1.5 inch needle that is fully inserted into the center of the testis and 10-15 ml of lignocaine hydrochloride instilled. The needle is withdrawn so that the tip is in a subcutaneous location, and 10 ml of anaesthetic is instilled on a line 1 cm from the median raphe from the cranial to caudal pole of the testis. The second testis is anaesthetized in the same manner. After anaesthetic infiltration, the surgeon should wait for 5 minutes for diffusion of the drug proximally into the spermatic cord. Many surgeons prefer to castrate horses using short-acting intravenous anaesthetics. A clean safe area to anaesthetize and recover the horse must be located. The horse is sedated with xylazine hydrochloride at 0.5-0.8 mg/kg IV. Ketamine hydrochloride 2.2 mg/kg and butorphanol tartrate 0.044 mg/kg are combined and given IV 5 minutes after xylazine administration. Duration of action of the anaesthetic combination is usually 10-15 minutes. If necessary, anaesthesia can be extended by administering half the dosage of xylazine and ketamine combined in one syringe.

Burdizzoo Castration

This is the most popular technique of castration in ruminants. In this technique, the spermatic cords with the blood vessels leading to the testicles are crushed. One

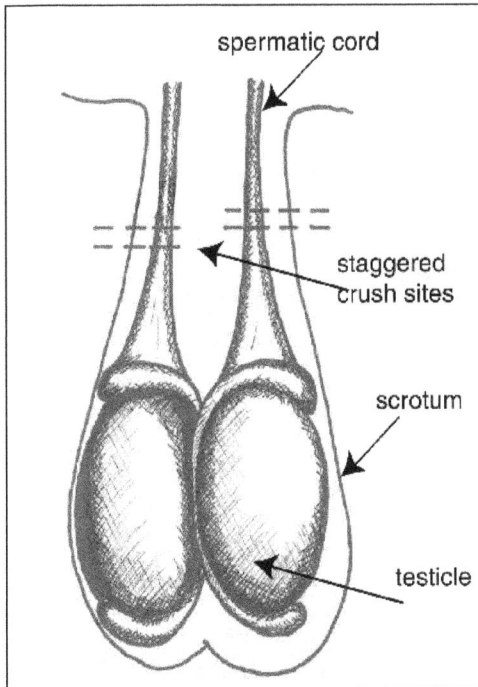

Figure 18.1: Burdizzo Castration Sites.

spermatic cord is clipped at a time and the two cords are clipped at different levels. Gradual atrophy of the testicles is noticed subsequently. Advantages of the technique are bloodless technique, less chances of infection (no open wounds), no risk of maggot infestation, less pain than cutting, and quickly and easily accomplished. Disadvantages include chances of injury to the animal and mistakes while clamping (penile trauma, crush site of the two sides meeting together arresting the blood supply to the scrotum thus resulting in gangrene and infection, slip of the cord from the crush or cord incompletely crushed).

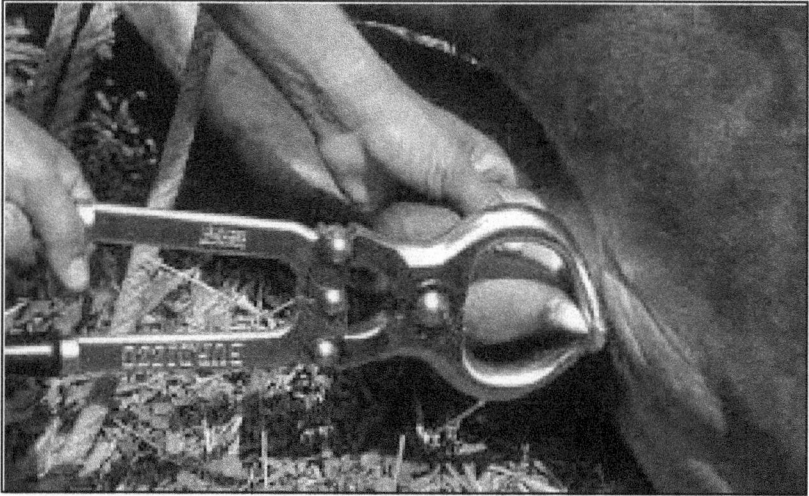

Figure 18.2: Castration of Cattle with Burdizzo Castrator.

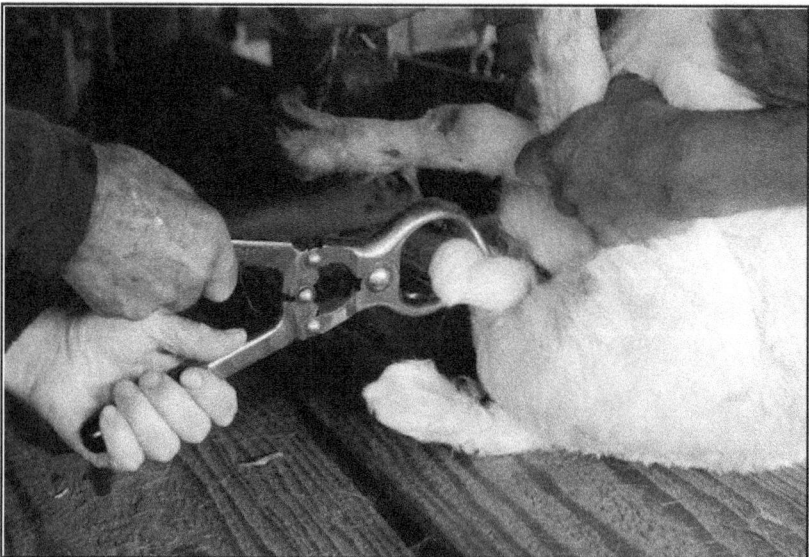

Figure 18.3: Burdizzo Castration in a Buck.

Elastrator

Castration is performed routinely in lambs during the first week after birth by applying tight rubber rings to the neck of the scrotum so that both testicles are below and two teats above the ring. Sloughing of the scrotum along with the testes distal to the ring generally takes three weeks time.

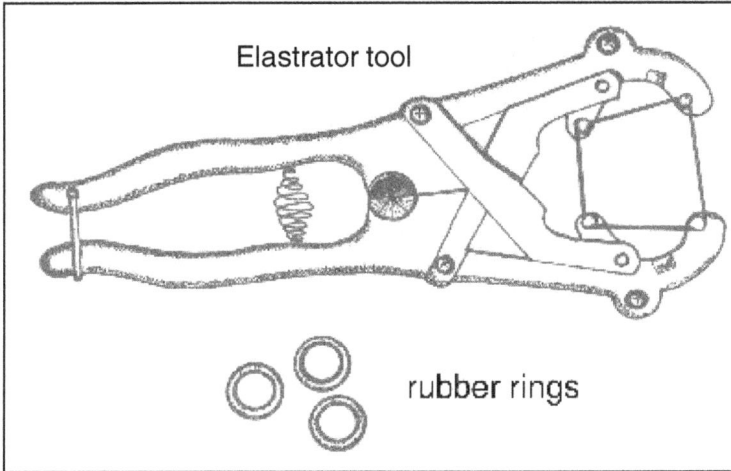

Elastrator tool

rubber rings

Figure 18.4: Elastrator Tool Used to Apply Rubber Rings.

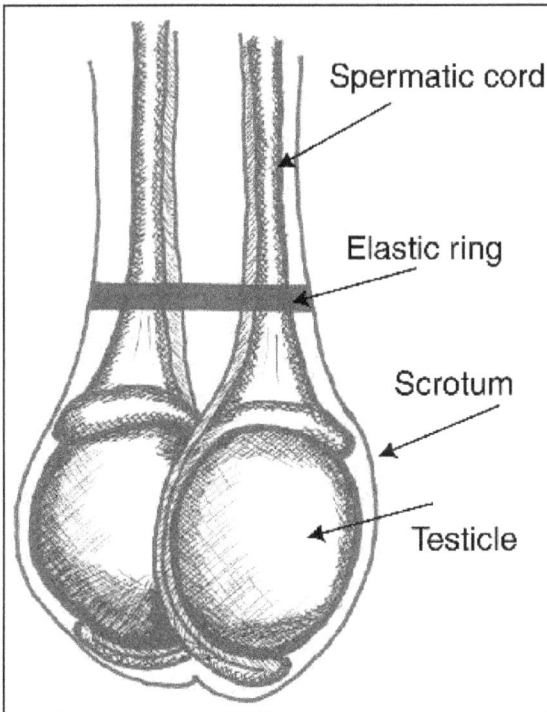

Spermatic cord

Elastic ring

Scrotum

Testicle

Figure 18.5: Elastic Band at Top of Testicles.

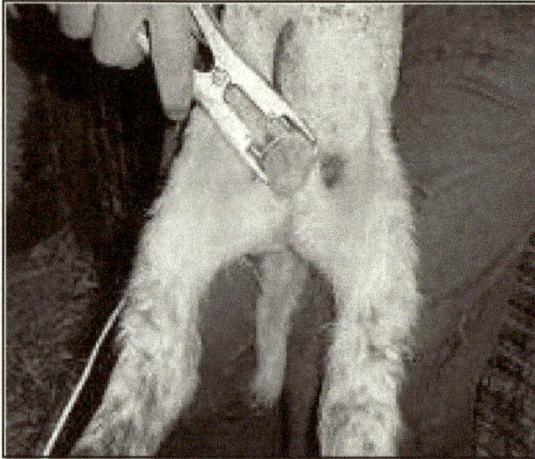

Figure 18.6: Lamb Castration with Elastrator.

Unilateral Orchiectomy

Valuable ruminants with nonheritable unilateral disorders other than herniation (hydrocele, haematocele, testicular tumour, epididymitis, abscess, varicocele) are subjected to unilateral orchiectomy. Vertical incision is made on the lateral aspect of the affected side of the scrotum approximately the entire length of the testis. Vaginal tunic is incised over the length of the testis. Spermatic cord is isolated, double ligated and transected or emasculated. The transected tunic is over sewn with an absorbable suture material. Excess scrotal skin is removed to reduce the dead space and prevent post-operative seroma formation. Scrotal fascia and skin are closed routinely.

In equines the castration technique involves orchiectomy, regardless of whether the horse is castrated while standing or recumbent. Scrotal incisions are given over each testis from cranial to caudal pole 1 cm parallel and away from the median raphe. The open technique of castration is probably the most commonly used technique. In this technique, the parietal (or common vaginal) tunic is retained. With the closed and the half-closed techniques, the portion of the parietal tunic that surrounds the testis and distal portion of the spermatic cord are removed. Routine castration is performed with an emasculator. The instrument crushes the spermatic cord to control haemorrhage, and severs the cord distal to the crushed area. For each technique, the emasculator is applied at a right angle to the spermatic cord, loosely closed to avoid incorporation of scrotal skin, and slid further proximally. The emasculator is applied in such a way that the crushing component is proximal to the cutting blade. When correctly applied, the wing-nut of the emasculator is oriented distally toward the testis, and the emasculator is positioned "nut to nut." Under field conditions the emasculotome is generally not available. The spermatic cord/vasculature can be carefully ligated using sterile nonabsorbable No.2 braided silk suture by transfixation proximal to the site of resection. By

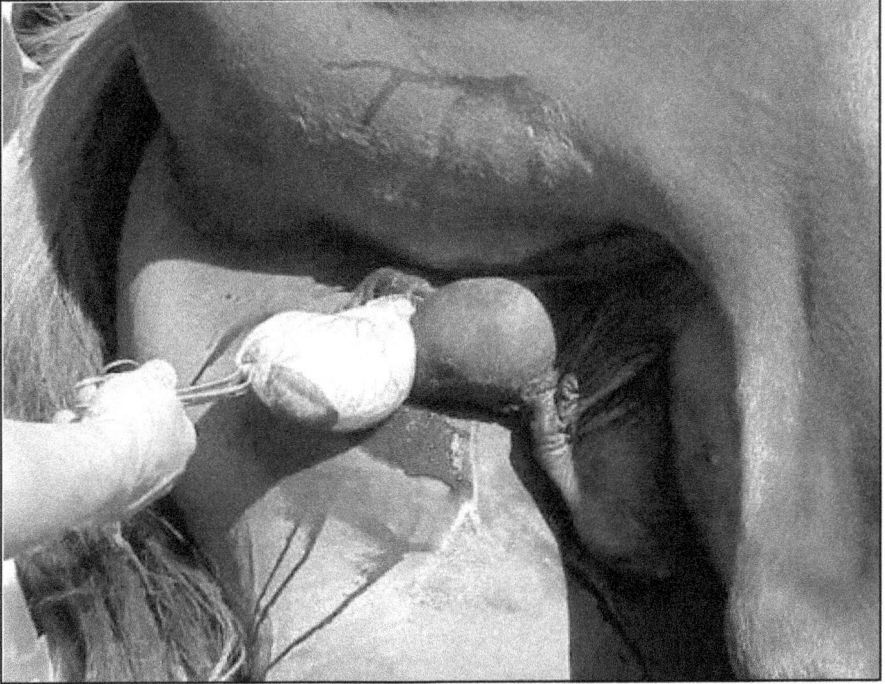

Figure 18.7: Open Castration of a Horse Performed in the Field Under a General Anaesthetic.

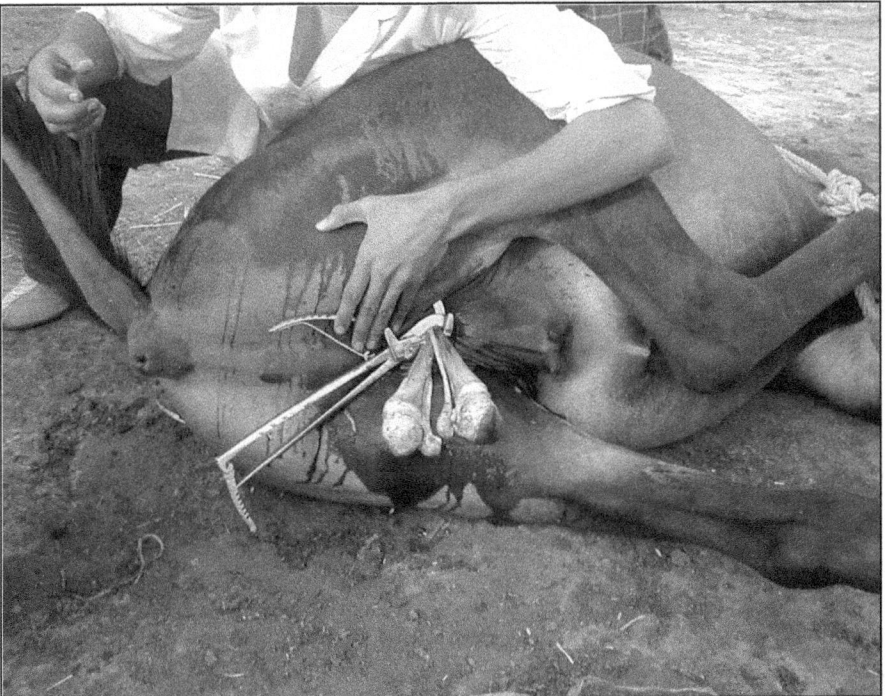

Figure 18.8: Use of Emasculotome during Equine Castration.

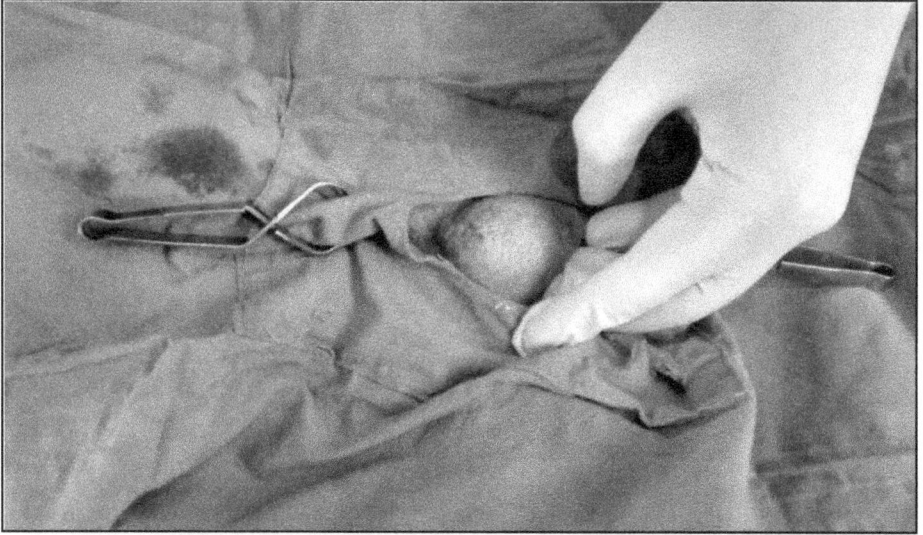

Figure 18.9: Testicle Pushed towards Pre-Scrotal before Castation

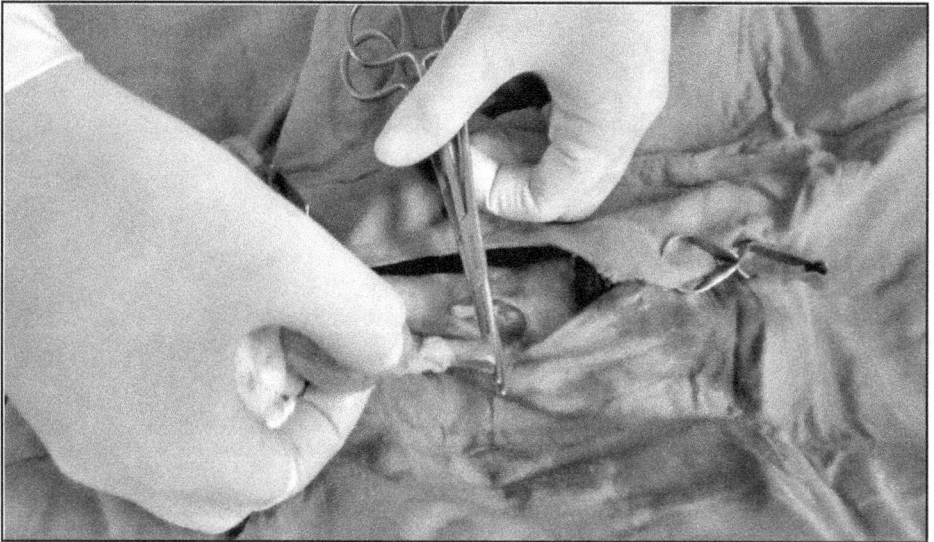

Figure 18.10: Canine Castration in Progress.

convention, scrotal incisions are usually left unsutured to heal by secondary intention. Primary closure, however, speeds up healing, and recovery eliminates infection and decreases oedema, pain and muscular stiffness. Primary closure may be particularly useful if vigorous exercise cannot be enforced post-operatively. Primary closure decreases convalescence but is time consuming and requires meticulous haemostasis and strict adherence to aseptic technique. All horses and small ruminants not previously immunized with tetanus toxoid are immunized.

The animal's activity is restricted for the first 24 hr after castration to avoid haemorrhage from the severed testicular and scrotal vessels. After this period, they are exercised to the degree necessary to prevent excessive preputial and scrotal oedema.

In the dog a median skin incision is made cranial to the scrotum and is carefully extended through the subcutaneous tissue layers. This incision should extend from the base of the scrotum a sufficient length cranially to allow expression of each testis through it. In dogs under 35 kg body weight, a closed castration technique is preferred. Large and giant breeds are castrated by the open method. In these animals, the testicular artery and vein, and the ductus deferens are collectively ligated with a suture proximal to the pampiniform plexus. The skin is carefully closed with a fine nonabsorbable suture material in an intracuticular or a simple interrupted pattern.

Pinhole Castration

Pinhole castration, an alternative simple, economical, quick, requiring no special instruments and field applicable technique, has recently been described in ruminants and stray dogs. Under sedation and local anaesthetic infiltration, *in situ* spermatic cord ligation is achieved by restraining the cord laterally within the scrotal

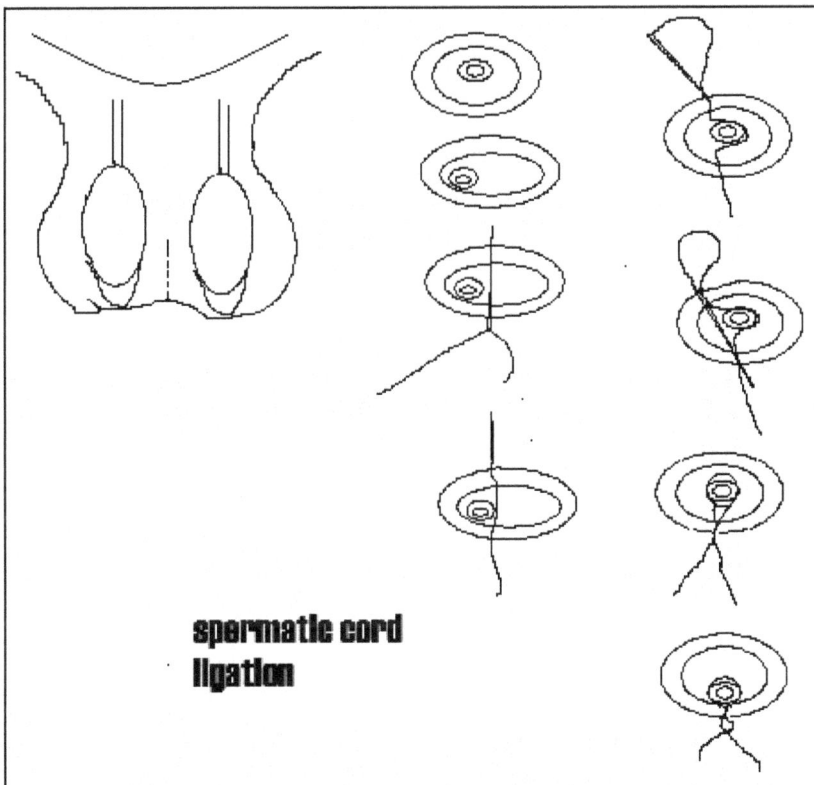

Figure 18.11: Pinhole Castration.

sac and passing catgut No. 1 through a hypodermic needle inserted caudal to cranial at the neck of the scrotum and adjacent to the medial margin of the restrained spermatic cord. The needle is removed leaving the suture in place and the spermatic cord repositioned medially. Then the needle is reinserted through the original holes, and the suture passed back through the needle. The hypodermic needle is subsequently withdrawn. The suture ends are tied to ligate the spermatic cord, leaving the square knot subcutaneously. Instead of the hypodermic needle, traumatic suture needle of a larger size or sterile silk may be used. The technique has high potential of managing large volume of stray dogs, monkeys and ponies in developing countries where the governments and the public may not afford comparatively expensive orchiectomy, the conventional procedure of castration. Strict asepsis and requirement of analgesics for 3 or more days following pinhole castration are the main disadvantages.

19

Ovariohysterectomy in Canines and Felines

A.K. Gangwar and Kh. Sangeeta Devi

Ovariohysterectomy is the surgical removal of the uterus and ovaries. It is a major surgical procedure which requires general anaesthesia, full theatre discipline and surgical technique. The uterus is an organ which comprises of a uterine body, two horns (to which the ovaries are attached) and a cervix. Strictly speaking the spaying of an animal means the removal of the ovaries (ovariectomy). When both ovaries and the uterus to the level of the cervix are removed this operation is known as an ovariohysterectomy.

Ovariohysterectomy is usually performed during anestrus, since reproductive and mammary tissues are more vascular under the influence of estrogen. Additionally, the uterus is more friable during estrus and may tear when crushed by clamps.

Indications

☆ *Elective sterilization*: Most common indication for ovariohysterectomy.

☆ *Heat prevention*: To prevent estrus and the associated problems such as bloody vaginal discharge, the nuisance of male dogs being attracted and unwanted pregnancies.

☆ *Treatment of ovarian and uterine diseases*: Ovariohysterectomy is indicated for the surgical treatment of ovarian cysts, pyometra, uterine torsion, uterine prolapse, uterine intussusceptions, uterine neoplasia and uterine rupture.

☆ *Mammary tumour reduction*: Spaying at an early age/before the first ovarian cycle reduces the risk and severity of mammary cancers. It is important to be aware that 50 per cent of mammary tumours are malignant in the entire (un-neutered) bitch.

☆ *Pyometra prevention*: Pyometra is an infection whereby the uterus fills with pus and the dog's condition deteriorates rapidly. It is a very serious condition, more commonly seen in the middle-aged and elderly bitch. Ovariohysterectomy is indicated as the treatment or prevention of pyometra.

☆ *Phantom pregnancy prevention*: Ovariohysterectomy is also indicated as a permanent treatment for recurrent and severe false pregnancy, phantom pregnancy or pseudocyesis. Phantom pregnancy may cause behavioural changes (*e.g.* depression, nest making) as well as physical changes (lactation, abdominal enlargement etc).

☆ To prevent recurrence of vaginal hyperplasia.

☆ To prevent hormonal changes that can interfere with medication in diabetic or epileptic dogs or cats.

Surgical Anatomy

☆ The ovaries are located ventral to the 4th lumbar vertebra and close to the caudal pole of the corresponding kidney.

☆ The ovary is completely enclosed by the bursa, except when it is enlarged by the ripe follicles at estrus.

☆ The ovary is attached to the cranial end of the uterine horn by the ovarian ligament, which is continuous with suspensory ligament of the ovary. The suspensory ligament is attached to the transverse fascia near the vertebral end of the last rib and offers the main resistance to withdrawal of the ovary from the abdomen.

☆ The blood supply to the ovary is through ovarian artery and vein. The artery leaves the aorta at 4th lumbar vertebra, crosses the caudal pole of the kidney and enters the dorsal curvature of the ovary.

☆ The uterus has two very long and narrow horns and a short body. The horns diverge from the body in the form of a 'V' towards each kidney.

☆ Broad ligament is attached to the anterior part of the vagina.

☆ Uterine artery originates from the urogenital artery and enters the caudal part of the broad ligament at the plane of the cervix and lies close to the caudal part of the uterus.

Surgical Procedure

Anaesthesia and Positioning of Animal

In field conditions the best anaesthetic combination is atropine-xylazine-ketamine (0.04 mg/kg, i.m. – 2 mg/kg, i.m. – 10 mg/kg, i.m.). Each drug should be given at an interval of 5 minutes. The animal can be maintained by giving extra dose of ketamine intravenously or diazepam @ 0.25 mg/kg, i.v. The animal is positioned in dorsal recumbency (midline approach) or right lateral recumbency (flank approach).

Aseptic Preparation of the Site

Mid-ventral area from the xephoid to pubis or lateral flank area is shaved and scrubbed with antiseptic solution. Finally betadine is painted at the site.

Approaches

The uterus and ovaries can be approached through one of the following techniques.

1. Midline incision approach
2. Flank incision approach
3. Laparoscopic technique

1. Midline Incision Approach

☆ The length of the midline abdominal incision is based on the species and size of the animal.

☆ The distance between the umbilicus and the pubis is divided into cranial, middle and caudal third.

☆ In dog, the incision is made in the cranial third because the ovaries are more difficult to exteriorize than the uterine body.

☆ In cat, the incision is made in the middle third because the uterine body is more difficult to exteriorize than the ovaries.

☆ The incision is made through the three layers to expose the abdominal contents (skin fascia- outer skin, linea alba-outer layer of muscle under the skin and peritoneum- inner muscle layer).

☆ The uterine horn is located by means of an ovariohysterectomy hook or the index finger.

☆ Apply a clamp on the proper ligament. The clamp is used to retract the ovary while the suspensory ligament is stretched or broken with the index finger.

☆ Make a window in the mesovarium caudal to the ovarian vessels. Three clamps are applied at the ovarian pedicle and the pedicle is severed between the clamp closest to the ovary and the middle clamp.

☆ The clamp applied distally from the ovary, is removed so that the pedicle ligature can be placed in its groove.

☆ The pedicle is ligated by chromic catgut.

☆ The pedicle is inspected for bleeding and gently replaced into the abdomen.

☆ Same procedure is repeated on the opposite ovarian pedicle.

☆ The blood vessels in the broad ligament can be ligated before severed or torn.

☆ Three clamps are placed on the uterine body just cranial to the cervix. The uterine body is severed between the proximal and middle clamps.

☆ The uterine arteries are individually ligated caudal to the most caudal clamp.

☆ Remove the caudal clamp and the uterus is ligated in the groove that remains.

☆ The pedicle is inspected for bleeding and gently replaced into the abdomen.

☆ At the end of surgery the abdominal incision is stitched up routinely in three layers. The outer layer of stitches on the skin fascia, if non-absorbable material is used, should be removed 10 days post-surgery.

☆ Immediate post-operative treatment generally includes pain relief, broad spectrum antibiotic, antiseptic dressing of the wound, exercise restriction and recovery diet. An Elizabethan collar is often given to prevent the dog from licking at the wound. Long term dietary modifications are often indicated to prevent obesity, which often occurs after spaying due to alteration in hormone levels.

Advantages

☆ Large ovarian tumours, and pyometra is best treated by this site

Disadvantages

☆ Incision size is large

☆ Chances of wound contamination, wound dehiscence and incisional hernia are more

☆ Wound healing is slow

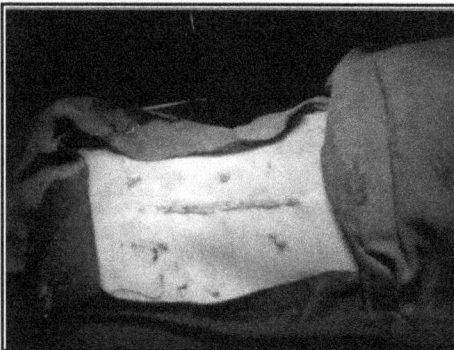

Figure 19.1: Mid Ventral Approach.

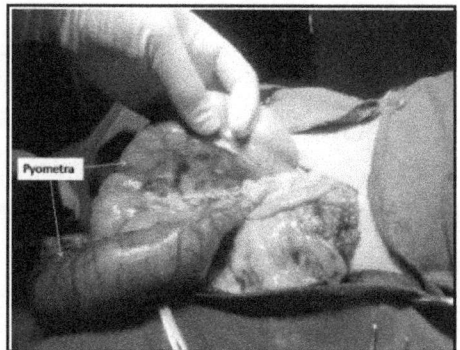

Figure 19.2: Ovariohysterectomy by Mid Ventral Approach.

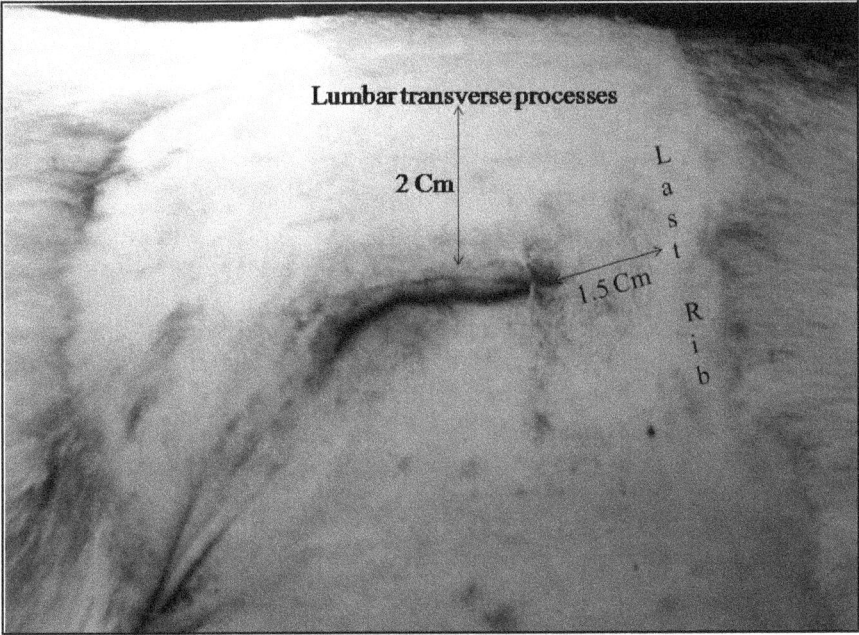

Figure 19.3: Flank Approach.

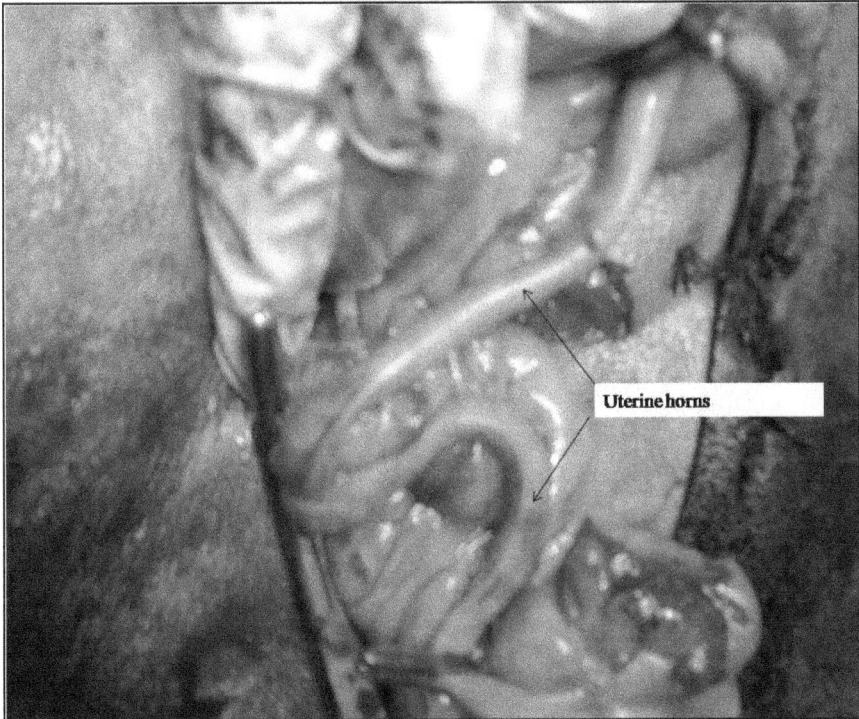

Figure 19.4: Ovariohysterectomy by Flank Approach.

2. Flank Approach

☆ Ovariohysterectomy through a single incision in the left flank is particularly useful in cats. However, right flank approach is preferred in bitches.

☆ The incision is usually located midway between the cranial aspect of the tuber coxae and the caudal most aspect of the last rib.

☆ The incision is usually made in a transverse plane and ranges from 2-8 cm in length. In bitches, obliquely downward and backward incision is made. After dissection through subcutaneous fat, a grid incision which involves blunt separation along the direction of the muscle fibers through the three muscular layers (abdominal external oblique, abdominal internal oblique, transversus abdominis) is made.

☆ Branches of the deep circumflex artery may be encountered with the transverse abdominal muscle layer and may require ligation. Alternatively, the layers may all be incised in a transverse plane instead of a grid.

Advantages

☆ Incision size is small

☆ Chances of wound contamination, wound dehiscence and incisional hernia are less

☆ Wound healing is fast

Disadvantages

☆ Large ovarian tumours and pyometra can not be treated by this site.

Complications

☆ Haemorrhage

☆ Ovarian remnant syndrome: due to the remnant of ovarian cells

☆ Uterine stump pyometra

☆ Inflammation and granuloma

☆ Fistulous tracks

☆ Ligation of ureter: accidental ligation of the ureter causing hydronephrosis or atrophy of the kidney

☆ Urinary incontinence

20

Caesarean Section

Rekha Pathak

Caesarean section is also commonly termed as C-section in which the uterus is exteriorized to take out the foetus from the pregnant dam.

Indications

- ☆ Uterine inertia
- ☆ Various types of obstructive dystocia (*e.g.*, emphysematous foetus, oversized foetus, small pelvic canal and pelvic fractures of the dam, and position and posture dystocia)
- ☆ Rupture of uterus (may be due to excessive manipulation of the foetus)
- ☆ Animal in highly compromised condition like pregnancy toxemia, weak prostrated dam unable to show labor etc.
- ☆ In the mares twin pregnancy is a common indication for C-section
- ☆ Uterine torsion
- ☆ Incomplete cervical dilatation

It is important to choose a clean and bright place for the operation. The air borne contamination should be strictly avoided and utmost care should be taken to prevent the post-operative complications and septicemia because the successful outcome of the operation is mainly dependent on the strict asepsis which is followed.

Site of the surgical operation varies with the type of species. In dogs the site is ventral line incision behind the umbilicus; in the cow a vertical or oblique incision on the left lower flank is preferred (for the reason that on the left side the intestinal

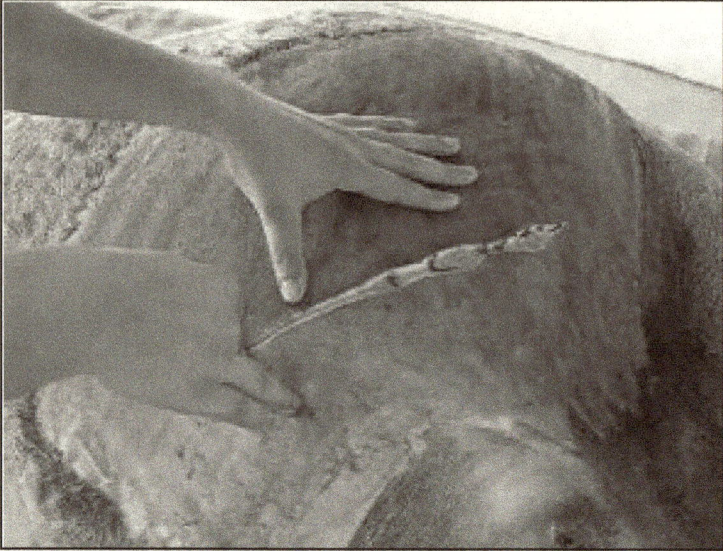

Figure 20.1: Left Lower Flank Incision in Cattle.

interference is least) (Figure 20.1). In mares, a left paramedian incision (caudal) or ventral midline incision is preferred. In small ruminants like goats and ewes, the sites chosen are just as in cattle. For left lower flank incisions, the animals are put on the right lateral recumbency, and for ventral midline incision they are put on the dorsal recumbency. It is important to comfortably cast the animal at an optimal height so that the surgeon is not only comfortable of his posture but since this operation takes relatively longer time and cumbersome, especially in large animals. There should be a skilled team consisting of at least two surgeons at the operative site and one assistant on the instrument table. Two skilled assistants should take care of the intravenous fluid administration and other drugs requirement of the casted animal. The animal should be first checked for dehydration and every attempt should be made for stabilizing the animal with administration of intravenous fluids and other life saving drugs like corticosteroids.

Surgical Anatomy

Dog

The gravid uterus has dilated horns in the shape of 'Y', which contains the foetuses and lies on the ventral abdominal floor extending up to the level of stomach towards the end of gestation.

Cow

The gravid uterus may lie directly up on the right abdominal floor or within the supraomental space with the intestine concealed on the right by superficial and deep parts of greaten omentum.

After giving an incision at the left lower flank, the uterus is usually brought outside by feeling and grasping the foetal parts. The uterus may be exposed for caesarean section by simply drawing the greater omentum forward. If the foetus in mummified, instead of giving a lower flank incision, upper flank incision is usually preferred; whereas in full term gestation because the uterus due to its weight is found on the ventral floor of the abdomen, it is better to go for the lower flank incision.

Anaesthesia

In dogs where the pups are found to be alive by ultrasonographic or Doppler examination, thiopental or xylazine is avoided for the reason of respiratory depression of pups, and a combination of epidural and local infiltration with 2 per cent Lignocaine can be given.

A combination of diazepam and ketamine can also be given intravenously at the dose rate of 0.5 mg/kg body weight and 5.0 mg/kg body weight, respectively. In cattle or buffalo, slight sedation may be needed sometimes along with local infiltration at the line of incision. In mares, inhalation anaesthesia with inhalant anaesthetic agents is preferred.

Surgical Technique

Midline incision behind the umbilicus includes incision on the ventral aponeurosis of the muscles (white line). The ventrolateral oblique incision is usually used in cows and buffaloes with the animals controlled in lateral recumbency and hind limbs extended caudally. Incision is made just in front of stifle extending cranioventrally in a slight oblique direction. The structures invaded are skin, subcutaneous fascia and combined aponeurosis of the two oblique muscles, which form the external sheath of the rectus abdominis, transverse abdominis and peritoneum. Paramedian incision is preferred in mares and the structures include skin, fascia, external rectus sheath, rectus abdominis muscle, internal rectus sheath and peritoneum.

Dogs can be premedicated with atropine sulfate @ 0.04 mg/kg body wt subcutaneously, followed by diazepam @ 0.5 mg/kg body wt and ketamine @ 2-5 mg/kg body wt. intravenously. This regimen is followed if the foetuses are found administered to be alive by other examinations. But if there is a certainty that foetuses are dead or infected, then atropine sulphate is followed by thiopentone sodium @ 8-10 mg/kg body wt. A long incision on the linea-alba is given in medium and small sized dogs to exteriorize the uterus. But if the animal's size is more than 25 kg an oblique incision is preferred on the flank or paramedian site to avoid post-operative dehiscence and hernia.

The cow is controlled in standing or right lateral recumbency and a long skin incision is given by saving the left subcutaneous abdominal vein. We can either give the local infiltration or epidural anaesthesia with 2 per cent lignocaine. In bitches, the bifurcation of uterine body is first visualized and an incision is made over it in order to enable the milking (squeezing) of pups from both the horns. The foetuses are removed along with foetal membranes one by one. The umbilical vessels are ligated and cut, and the new born foetuses are handed over to a helper or nurse for resuscitation. They are wiped with mops and assisted for artificial respiration if fail to breathe. The head is lowered to permit drainage of fluids from the upper respiratory tract. In cow the uterine incision should follow the longitudinal line of greater curvature of the uterus.

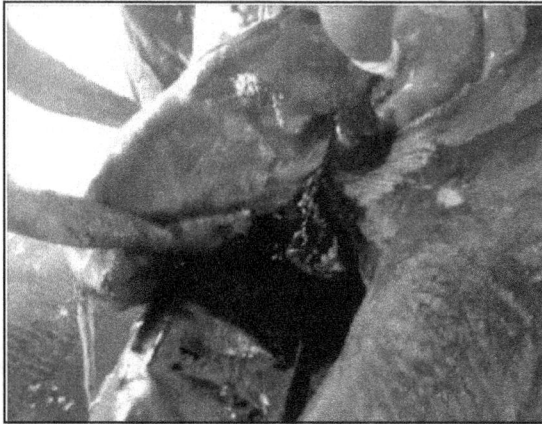

Figure 20.2: Foetus being Taken Out from the Uterus.

Forelimbs or hind limbs are grasped depending upon the presentation and the foetus is taken out from the uterus (Figure 20.2). The calf should be taken care by the assistants. It should be cleaned, dried, cleared off the mucus from the nostrils. The umbilical cord is ligated far enough from the navel and cut so that it contracts. Antiseptic solution like povidone iodine or tincture iodine is then applied over it to prevent any infection.

The removal of after-births or placenta is also important. If it is easily removed by gentle traction it should be removed, and it should not be pulled with force since chances of caruncular bleeding is strong, which may be fatal to the dam. If such bleeding is encountered in the dam, oxytocin should be given, which largely shrinks the uterus and stops bleeding. Antibiotics can be instilled into the uterus as common procedure for all the species before closure. The uterine incision is cleaned with a gauze and closed by a double row of Lamberts cushing sutures using chromic catgut size 2-0 or 3-0 in bitch and size 2 or 3 in cattle and buffaloes. Abdominal incisions are sutured in routine manner, closing the peritoneum, muscles and skin, respectively (Figures 20.3 and 20.4).

Utmost care is taken to avoid the spillage of uterine contents into the peritoneal/ abdominal cavity for the successful outcome of surgery. In case such spillage occurs, the abdominal cavity should be lavaged with sterile normal saline containing non-irritant antibiotics to counteract the infection, reduce the chances of post-operative adhesions and infection. The uterine torsion in case of cattle and buffaloes should be then corrected. Administration of 50-60 units of oxytocin hastens the uterine involution. Intravenous administration of a 5 per cent solution of dextrose or normal saline should be invariably included in the schedule as most deaths occur due to hypoglyacemia and hypochloraemia.

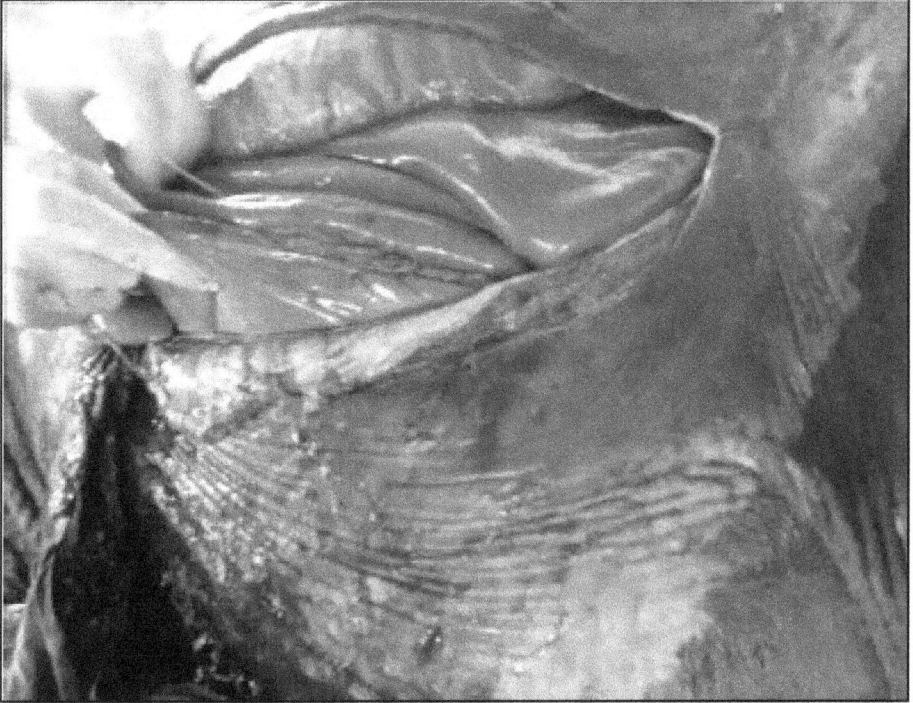
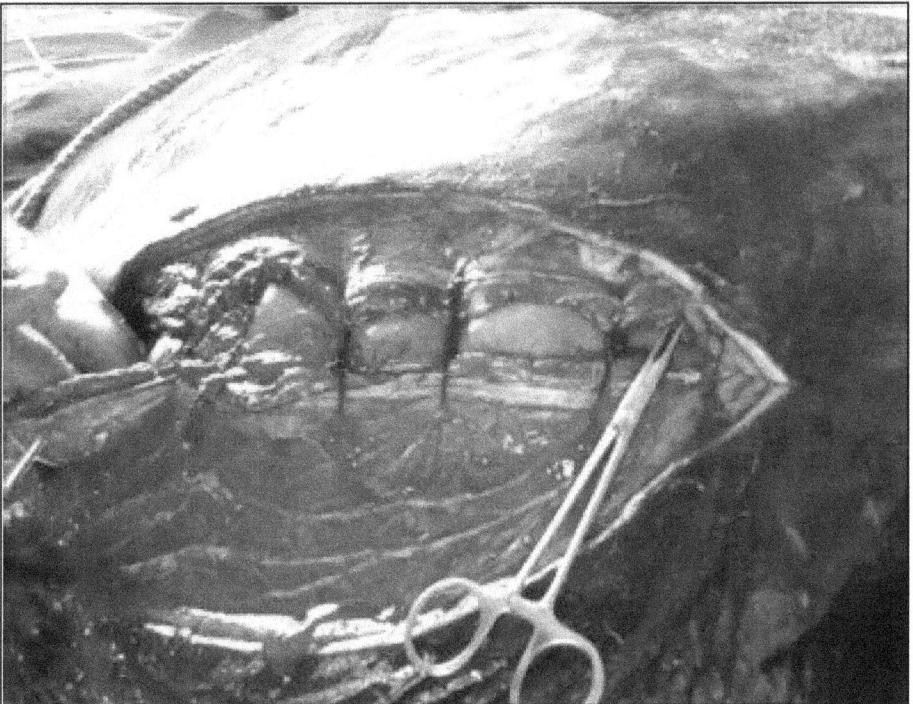

Figures 20.3 and 20.4: Closure of Uterine and Abdominal Incisions.

Post-operative Care

The mother and the new born foetus should be returned to clean and comfortable environment. If the haemorrhage is excessive, pituitrin and calcium gluconate may be given intravenously in bitches. Penicillin or some other antibiotics should be given. If the condition of the patient is poor, administration of blood or plasma expanders and corticosteroids is considered.

Puppies should be given to the mother as soon as she is ready to take care of them. Similarly the new born calf should also be allowed to suckle and stand on its legs. It not only provides the nourishment to the puppies but will also stimulate the uterine contractions thereby reducing any risk of placental retention or endometritis. The skin sutures should be removed in 10-12 days after surgery or after the healing is complete.

21

Management of Fractures

Hari Prasad Aithal

Fracture is a break in the continuity of bone. Fractures are common in animals and are caused either by direct trauma like automobile accidents or by indirect trauma caused while running, jumping or falling from a height. Fracture may also be caused by violent muscle contractions or by systemic/metabolic diseases like rickets or osteomalacia, wherein the bone becomes weak leading to fracture.

Based on the communication of fracture site with the environment, it can be classified as *simple (closed)* fracture or *compound (open)* fracture. Based on the extent of fracture line, it can be classified as *incomplete* or *complete* fracture. Based on the direction of fracture line in relation to the longitudinal axis of bone, fracture can be called as *transverse, oblique, spiral, comminuted* (more than two bone fragments) or *multiple* (two or more independent fractures of the same bone). Based on the location of fracture, it can be classified as *diaphyseal, metaphyseal or epiphyseal fracture.*

Diagnosis of Fracture

Diagnosis of a bone fracture is relatively easy. The first sign of a fracture is generally a non-weight bearing lameness. The fracture site shows signs of swelling, and the animal carry the affected leg, though it can move on three legs. Incomplete fractures, sometimes, are difficult to detect, as they usually cause only mild lameness. Confirmative diagnosis of a fracture can be done by radiographic examination. Generally both medio-lateral and cranio-caudal or dorso-plantar/dorso-palmar views are indicated. In recent years digital X-ray has increased the accuracy of diagnosing a fracture. Modern diagnostic methods like digital X-ray, CT scan, nuclear scintigraphy and MRI are particularly useful, where sometimes a survey radiograph fails to diagnose a fracture. However, these advanced diagnostic tools are generally beyond the reach of a common veterinary practitioner at the field level.

First Aid

First aid and careful handling of the animal before definite fracture fixation is important in veterinary practice. The animal should not be forced to walk on the broken leg or transported to the hospital without a proper splint, to avoid a relatively simple fracture becoming a comminuted or compound fracture. The animal must be restricted from moving on three legs to reduce further damage to the surrounding soft tissues, blood vessels and nerves. Fractured limb should be stabilized first by applying splint, which allows the animal to regain control of the leg even though it can not put complete weight on it. In excited animals it may be necessary to sedate the animal for splinting. A rigid splint (any lightweight, relatively strong, rigid material, such as wood or PVC pipe split lengthwise) is placed over the layer of cotton role applied over the skin and wrapped with a cotton/elastic bandage. Splint should not be used directly against the animal's skin. At least two pieces of wood/PVC tubing must be placed 90° apart (never 180°), one along the outer surface and the other along the front or the back of the leg. Placing

Figure 21.1: Radiograph Showing Comminuted Fracture at the Proximal End of Metatarsus in a Cattle.

the splint along the inner and outer surface of the leg is ineffective, as it does not prevent the leg from bending.

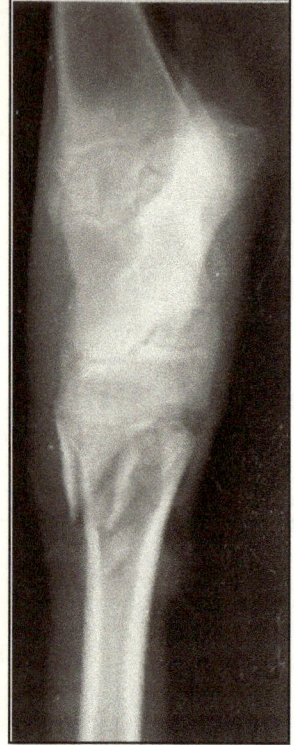

Factors to be Considered Before Fracture Fixation

The outcome of a fracture and fracture fixation depends on many factors that vary from case to case. Many animals with simple fractures recover with rest and proper care. Others with much more serious injuries have to undergo surgical fixation at the earliest. Early care and fracture fixation to stabilize the bone fragments is essential to minimize fracture complications. Several factors that should be considered while selecting the technique of fracture management, like, age, body weight and species of the animal, location and type of fracture, presence or absence of soft tissue and neuromuscular trauma, closed or open fracture environment, ability of the animal to stand and walk, and behavioural nature of the animal, the facilities available and above all the experience of the surgeon with a particular technique. The cost of treatment is also a major concern in veterinary practice.

External Fixation Techniques

External fixation refers to immobilization of fractures/other skeletal

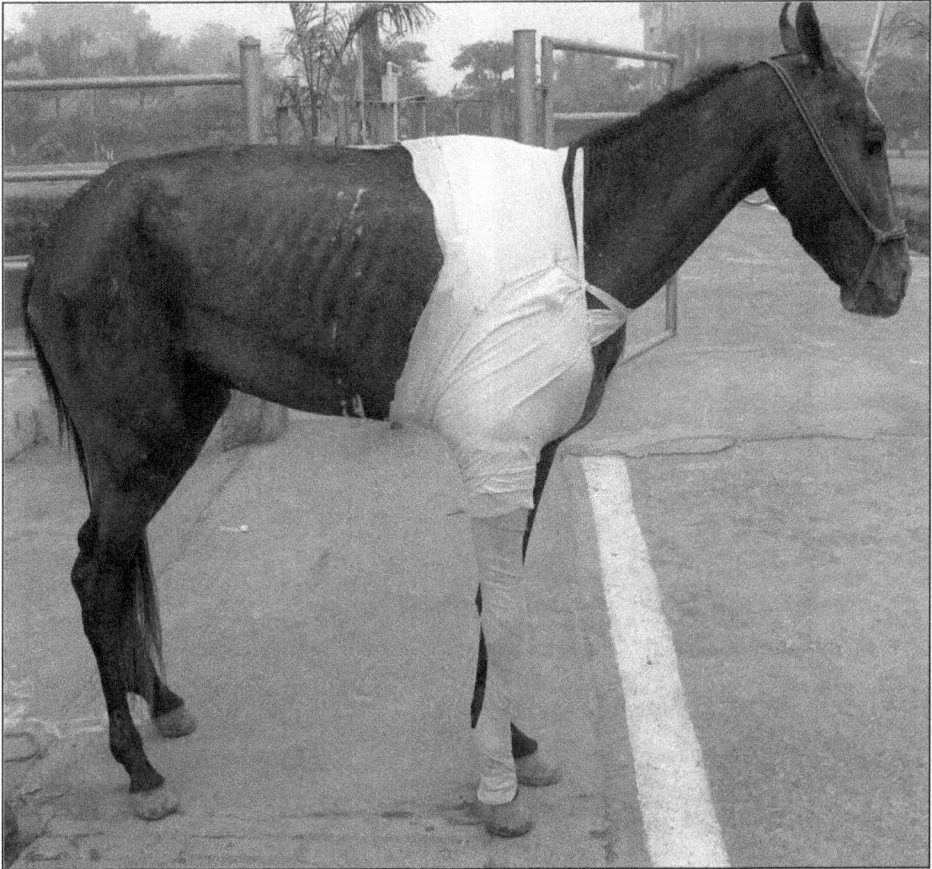

Figure 21.2: A Horse with Scapular Fracture Treated with Conservative Method.

abnormalities with devices applied externally, without the use of any invasive technique. Among the external fixation devices, plaster of Paris and modified Thomas splints are widely used.

Plaster Cast

Plaster bandages consist of a cotton bandage that has been impregnated with plaster pf Paris, which hardens after it has been made wet. It is the most widely used external fixation technique in both small and large animals. Indicated in immobilization of fractures below the mid-diaphysis of radius or tibia. The animal is restrained under sedation/anaesthesia. The placement of the cast is facilitated by use of rope restraint. An assistant should help to maintain alignment of the limb during application, being sure to check the position of the limb in cranio-caudal and latero-medial planes. In large animals, the tension on the limb during casting may be achieved by placing wires through holes drilled in the hoof wall and applying tension. The talcum powder may be sprinkled over the limb and an even layer of cotton is applied around the leg in order to protect bony prominences.

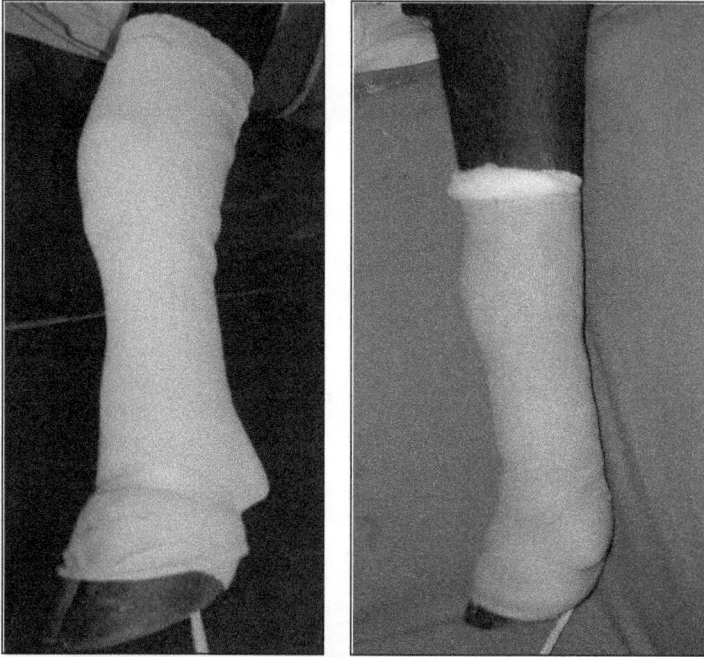

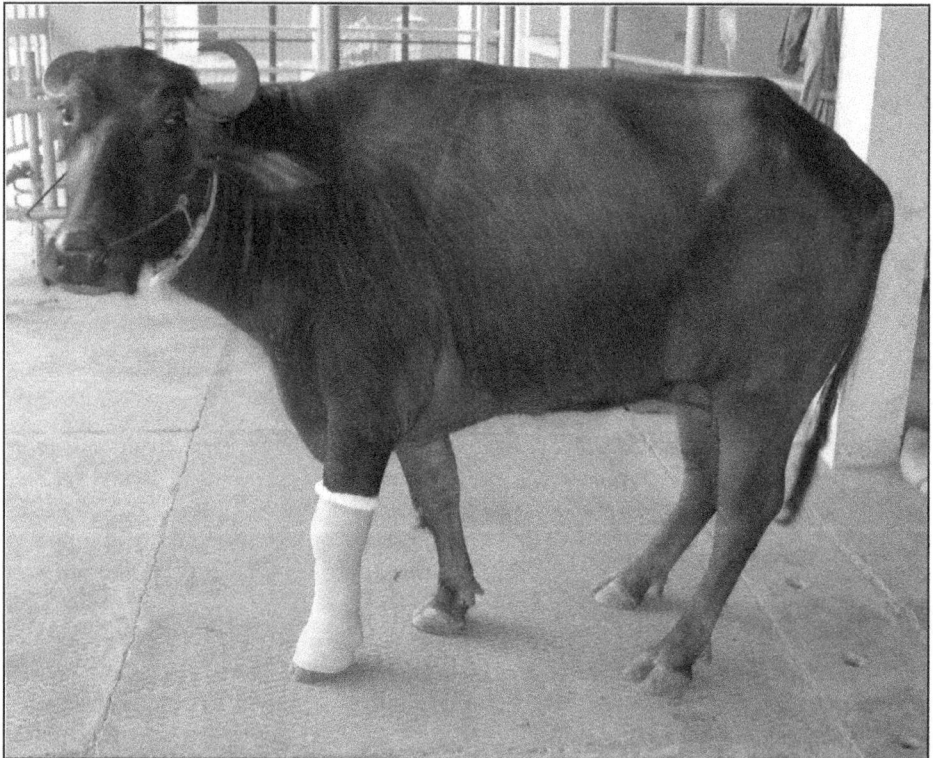

Figure 21.3: Technique of Fiberglass Casting.

Over padding should be avoided because it may impair immobilization by allowing movement of fracture fragments within the cast. Splints are bandaged in place with an even pressure. Plaster of Paris bandage is soaked in warm water for a few seconds until air bubbles cease to appear. Plaster bandage is then removed from the water, squeezed and wrapped over the splints, starting at the fracture site and continuing up and down including the entire limb except the toe pads in dogs and hooves in large animals. The plaster cast is never stretched or tightened around the limb. The plaster is moulded by rubbing each section with wet hand before the plaster is set. The thickness of the cast is usually based on clinical judgement. Casts 4-5 layers thick may be adequate for small animals, 6-8 layers for calves less than 150 kg body weight, but adult cattle may require 12-16 layers thick casts. Casts used on the hind limbs must be thicker because of stress concentration by the angulation of the hock. Incorporation of splints (wooden/metal) within the cast (2 rods placed 90° to each other) will increase the strength of the cast. The plaster is then allowed to dry and harden. Complete drying/hardening of the cast (attaining full strength) may take 24-72 hrs. Use of a walking bar ('U' shaped bar placed under the hoof and incorporated into the cast) will increase the distribution of loading forces into the cast and away from the distal limb. In open fractures, a window should be left at the site of wound for drainage and regular dressing.

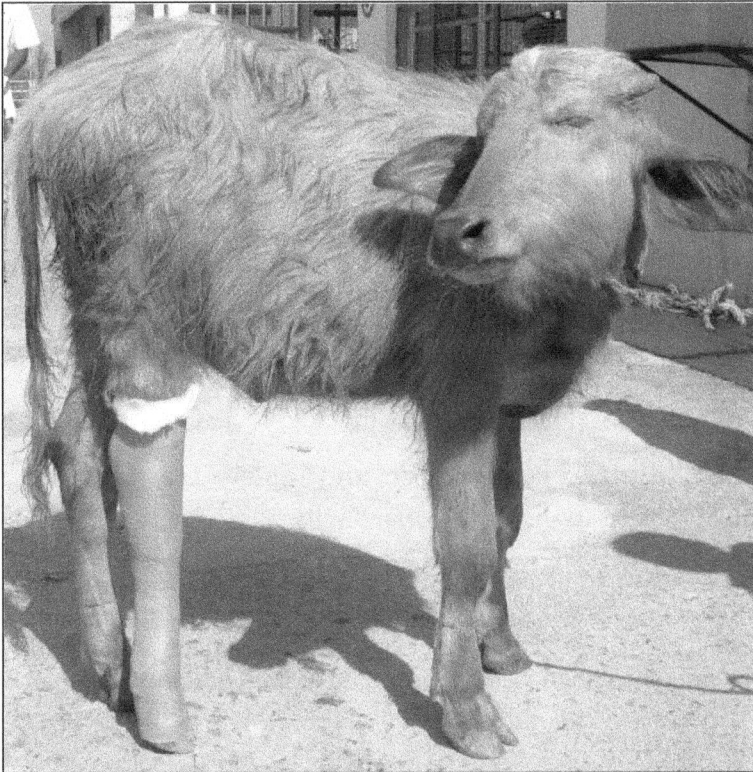

Figure 21.4: A Buffalo Calf with Metatarsal Fracture Treated with Fibre Glass Application.

Toes and hooves are inspected several times during the first 24 hr for any swelling, coldness or constriction. If the toe/hoof gets swollen or gets cold, pressure at the end of the cast should be relieved by removing the cast and the cast may be reapplied after swelling subsides. Cast may be maintained for up to 3-4 weeks in young dogs, 4-6 weeks in adult dogs and calves. Fractures in adult cattle may heal within 8-10 weeks, but often require 12-16 weeks for clinical union to occur. Plaster is removed after radiographic fracture union (bony union with resolution of the fracture line) takes place. Affected limb is massaged to promote circulation after removal of the cast. Movement is restricted till the limb regains its normal function.

Fiberglass cast is a lighter, synthetic alternative to the more traditional plaster cast. It is created by padding the extremity with cotton or waterproof padding material, followed by wrapping several layers of knitted fiberglass bandages impregnated with a water-soluble, quick-setting resin. It is lighter and more durable than plaster, so fiberglass has quickly become the preferred type of casting with many practitioners. Though it is slightly more costly, it is easily available everywhere and can be easily practised in the field level.

The fiberglass cast has many advantages over a plastic cast. It weighs less and is more comfortable. It is made of water-activated polyurethane resin combined with bandaging materials, so this material offers greater strength and less time for setting. A fiberglass cast requires less maintenance than a plaster cast. The fiberglass cast is waterproof. Some of the drawbacks with fiberglass cast are: it sets quickly, so a less-experienced medical care provider has less time to properly wrap the injured extremity. Further, the synthetic materials leave less room for swelling, and knitted fiberglass and resin bandages are less moldable than the plaster cast.

Modified Thomas Splints

Modified Thomas splint is indicated for immobilization of fractures at the distal femur, radius/ulna, distal humerus and tibia/fibula. The splint can be prepared from aluminum rods or conduit pipes of various sizes. For fore limbs, the length of the bar should be the distance from the thigh up to the tip of the toe in an extended leg. To prepare the ring, a splint mold is used and the rod is bent around the splint mold. The use of Thomas splint and cast combination is appropriate for fractures distal to the elbow or stifle in large animals.

External Skeletal Fixation Techniques

External skeletal fixation (ESF) refers to the stabilization of musculoskeletal injury using percutaneous fixation pins that are connected outside the body to form a rigid frame or scaffold, spanning the region of instability, *e.g.* transfixation pinning and casting, and different linear and circular fixators. This type of fixation is indicated for the management of long bone fractures especially of tibia and radius, where cast immobilization is not appropriate or does not provide optimal level of fixation (fractures proximal to the distal radial or tibial physis, with soft tissue injuries and open fractures).

Advantages of ESF include early return to function of the affected limb with excellent mechanical properties, ability to adjust the frame after bone fixation

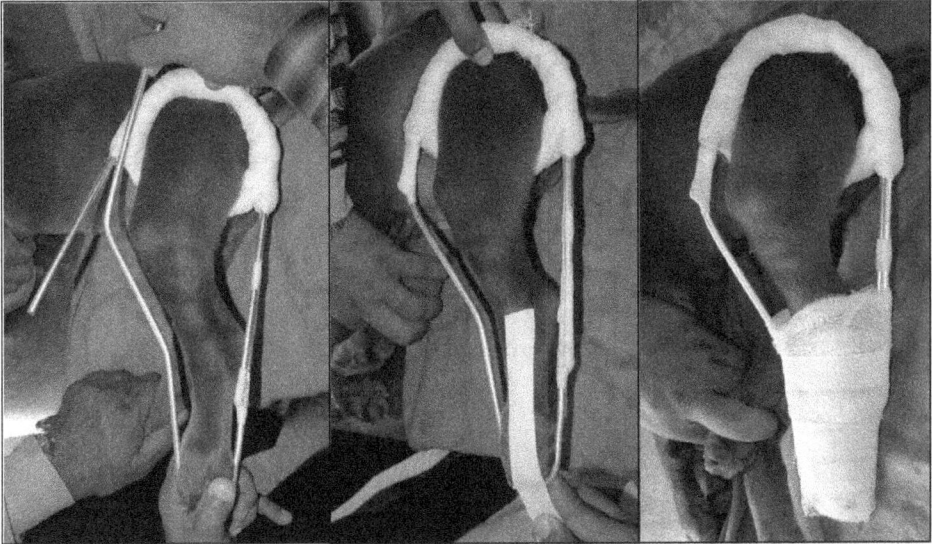

Figure 21.5: Application of Modified Thomas Splint in a Dog.

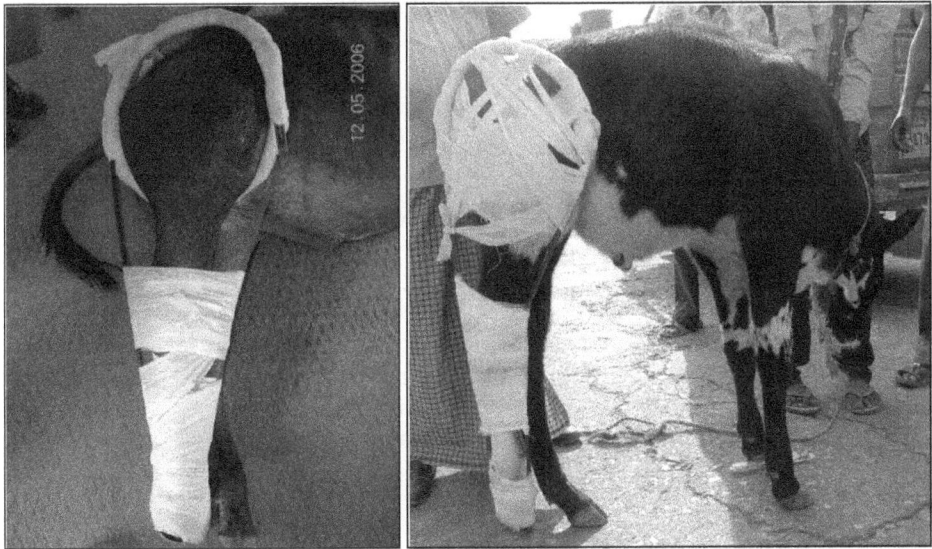

Figure 21.6: Modified Thomas Splint for Fixation of Femoral Fracture in Calves.

allowing correction of rotational or angular deformities, avoidance of surgical trauma to the injured tissue, avoidance of infection associated with buried implants, ease of implant removal after fracture union, provision for transarticular fixation in the presence of severe soft tissue trauma or severe comminution of the proximal or distal end of the affected bone, preservation of joint motion and multiple applications with reusability of components.

Transfixation Pinning and Casting

Transfixation pinning and casting (TPC) may be applied either as a "hanging limb pin cast" or as external skeletal fixator. Hanging limb pin cast refers to placement of transcortical/transfixation pins through the bone proximal to the injury, followed by application of a full limb cast. This avoids the slippage of cast, especially in hind limbs. The advantage of using pin-casts for ESF (where pins are passed both in the proximal and distal bone fragments) compared with hanging limb casts is that the fracture is more stable and the fracture fragments are not able to move within the pin-cast, and the pin-cast may not need to span adjacent joints in large animals. These techniques can easily be practised under field conditions with least instrumentation and technical support.

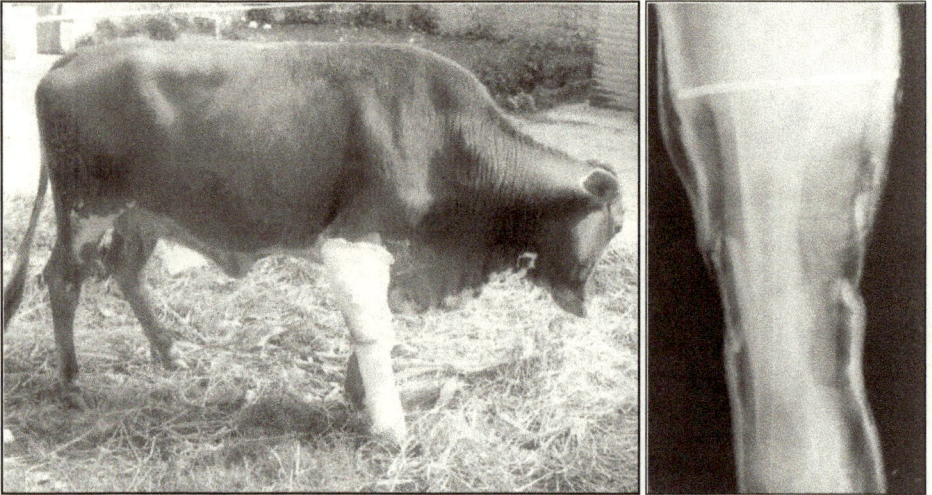

Figure 21.7: TPC for Fixation of Radial Fracture in an Adult Heavy Animal.

For management of open fractures, daily dressing of the wound may be carried out by leaving a hole in the cast (window cast) at the site of injury. However, this gives unsatisfactory access to the wound and is uncomfortable to the patient because the swelling in the limb becomes concentrated at the defect in the cast. Alternatively, metal or acrylic side bars may be used; they must be large enough to sustain the weight of the animal.

Acrylic and Epoxy-Pin Fixation Systems

This is a novel technique of fixation, where materials like acrylic (eg, polymethyl-methacrylate) and epoxy putty (M-seal) are used to construct the exernal frame of the fixator. Advantages of this free form fixation includes contouring the connecting bars to match any fracture configuration, pin direction need not be influenced by connecting bar location, and pin diameter need not be influenced by clamp size. Free form fixators have been generally used for mandible and maxilla fractures in dogs and for fractures of small bones in birds. But in recent years, they have been found effective for management of open long bone fractures in dogs,

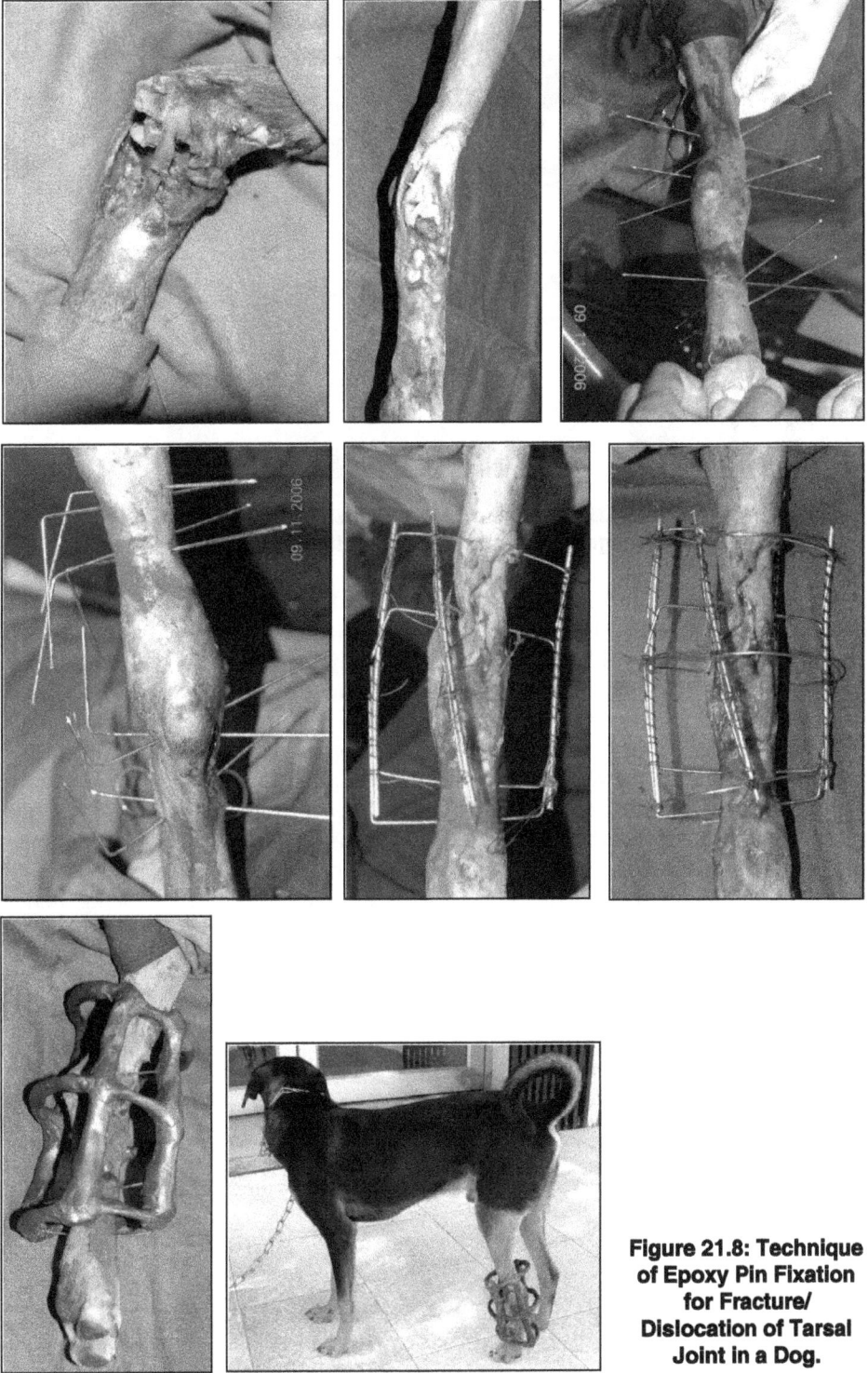

Figure 21.8: Technique of Epoxy Pin Fixation for Fracture/ Dislocation of Tarsal Joint in a Dog.

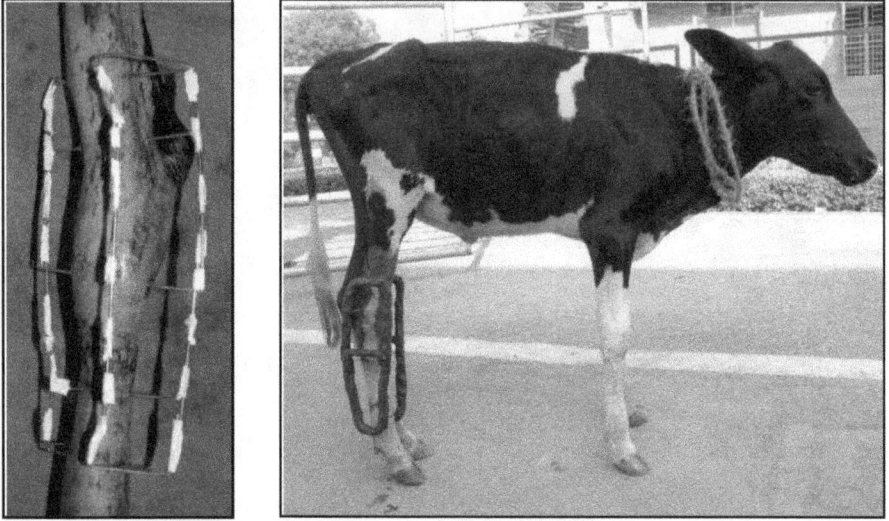

Figure 21.9: Epoxy-Pin External Skeletal Fixation for Management of Metatarsal Fracture in a Calf.

sheep/goats, calves and foals. They can be used for repair of open fractures/dislocations distal to the stifle and elbow joints. Fractures/dislocations are reduced and immobilized using 1.2-2.5 mm K-wires fixed at different levels (at least at 2 points in each fragment). Fixation wires in the same plane are bent and joined; and using additional wires, connecting bars/rings are constructed to make a temporary scaffold. Thoroughly mixed epoxy putty is then applied using the scaffold as guide and by incorporating the wires within the epoxy mold. In acrylic systems, the fixator components are constructed using acrylic columns with the use of flexible hollow plastic pipes, which are attached to the fixation pins. The fixation of acrylic/epoxy-pin ESF is easy, less cumbersome, needs minimal instrumentation, economical and also provides stable fixation of fractures in animals weighing up to 100 kg, hence can be practiced by a veterinary surgeon at any remote corner in the field.

22

Tendon Surgery

A.M. Pawde

The tendons are important constituents of the musculo-skeletal system through which the energy is transmitted, channelised, distributed and expressed in the form of movements. They are dense, irregular collagenous tissues composed of fibroblasts, parallel collagen fibres embedded in a ground substance.

Tendon Morphology

Tendon is composed of water (approx 70 per cent) and dry matter (30 per cent -collagen and non-collagenous matrix).

Collagen

Type I: most prevalent

Type II: within enthesious insertion and where tendon changes its direction.

Types III, IV and V: basement membranes and endotenon

Non-Collagenous Substances

Composed of tenocytes and glycoproteins

Tenocytes: (type I, II and III)

I and II – higher metabolic activity – concerned with extracellular matrix synthesis.

Glycoproteins

Cartilage oligomeric matrix protein (COMP)-most abundant-accumulated more in high load bearing tendons (flexors) than low load bearing tendons (extensors)-plays structural role.

Proteoglycans: Consist of Glycosaminoglycan

- ☆ Chondroitin sulphate
- ☆ Dermatan sulphate
- ☆ Keratan sulphate
- ☆ Heparin sulphate
- ☆ Heparin
- ☆ Hyaluronic acid

(More at metacarpo-phalangeal region than mid metacarpal-reflect functional and metabolic variance that exists between regions of tension and compression)

Smaller Proteoglycans

Decorin (lacking-results in large irregular collagen fibrils with poor mechanical strength)

Fibromodulin

Biglycan

(throughout the tendon-influence tenocyte function, collagen fibrillogenesis, spatial organisation of collagen fibres-tendon strength)

Outstanding feature of a normal tendon is its ability to glide through the surrounding tissue. All tendons have basic physical characteristics of tensile strength, compactness and smooth surface. Tendons are more prone to injuries due to their superficial location in the body.

Tendon injuries are more common in equines as compared to bovines.

Most Commonly Affected Tendon to Injury

Equine – SDF tendon (metacarpal region)

Bovines – SDF and DDF tendons, gastrocnemius and peroneus tertius.

Canines – SDF, DDF, extensors of fore paw and common calcanean tendon

Two major problems encountered in tendon reconstruction

- ☆ Formation of gap between the cut ends of the tendon
- ☆ Adhesions with peritendinous structures after surgical repair

Tendonitis

Etiopathology

Physical: fatigue, poor conformation, lack of exercise, incordinated muscle activity-degenerative changes, exercise induced hyperthermia (45°C)-damage to matrix.

Vascular. ischaemia, reperfusion injury, fibroblast anoxia.

Diagnosis

- ☆ Ultrasonography: most common technique used to diagnose tendonitis and monitor tendon healing
- ☆ Tendon/lesion cross sectional area
- ☆ Lesion type
- ☆ Location
- ☆ Fibre alignment
- ☆ Change in echogenecity
- ☆ Serological markers: COMP and others.

Treatment

Physical

- ☆ Ice application
- ☆ Bandaging
- ☆ Box rest
- ☆ Physiotherapy:
- ☆ Active/passive exercise

Pharmacological

- ☆ Anti-inflammatory drugs- in early period (less than 24 hrs)
- ☆ Sodium hyaluronate-intralesional/peritendinous
- ☆ Polysulphated glycosaminoglycans (PSGAGs)-inhibit macrophage activation, collagenase activity, metalloproteinase-in acute stage and later on- improve collagen fibril organization and stimulate tenocytes to produce collagen
- ☆ Beta-aminoproprinitrile fumerate (BAPM-F)- found in seed of Lathyrus odoratus (sweet pea), binds enzyme lysyl oxidase-inhibit deamination of lysin.

Surgical

- ☆ AL-SDFT desmotomy
- ☆ Percutaneous tendon splitting
- ☆ Counterirritation: topical blister ointments/line firing/pin firing (increase vascularity/inflammatory cell exudate).

Miscellaneous

- ☆ Low intensity ultrasound
- ☆ Low frequency infrared laser therapy
- ☆ Electro-magnetic field therapy.

Principles of Tendon Surgery

☆ Anaesthesia- deep sedation and local infiltration in large animals

☆ To minimize post-operative adhesion formation, skin incisions should not be given directly over the tendon

☆ The skin incision should be either parallel to the proposed site or curved over the tendon or curvilinear, so that healing skin wounds does not adhere to the tendon repair (tenorrhaphy) site

☆ Haemostasis should be complete

☆ All tissues should be handled gently

☆ The tendon should be kept moist with sterile saline and should not be allowed to become dry

☆ Skin hooks or hypodermic needles may be used for holding the tendon

☆ Suture materials for tenorrhaphy- ideal suture material should provide firm anchorage, produce a minimum of disruption and avoid burdening of tissue

☆ Suture material used for tendon surgery are nylon, polypropylene, polyethylene, polyester, stainless steel, silk, polydioxanone and polyglycolic acid (Vicryl).

Tendon Suturing Techniques

Bunnell Technique

Two needles on a single thread are used. Needle enters the tendon transversely 1 cm from the cut end and again at 45 degree pointing towards the cut end. One loop is placed in each segment and knot tied on the outside of one segment.

Bunnell-Mayer Technique

A transverse stitch is placed in both the cut ends of the tendon. The knots are tied at the cut ends of tendon. Advantage-round and semi round tendons are repaired more effectively; Disadvantage-not suitable for small flat tendons.

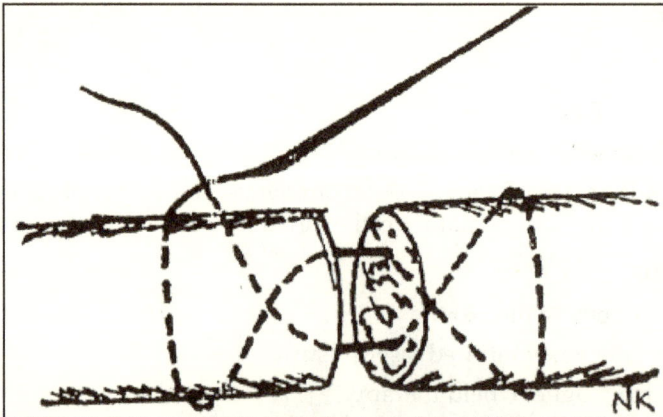

Figure 22.1

Modification of Bunnell Technique

Procedure is repeated as in Bunnell technique but instead of one loop, two loops are placed in each segment.

Locking Loop Technique (Kessler-Mason Technique)

Have two components-longitudinal and transverse. To tighten loop on tendon fibres, the transverse component should be superficial over the longitudinal.

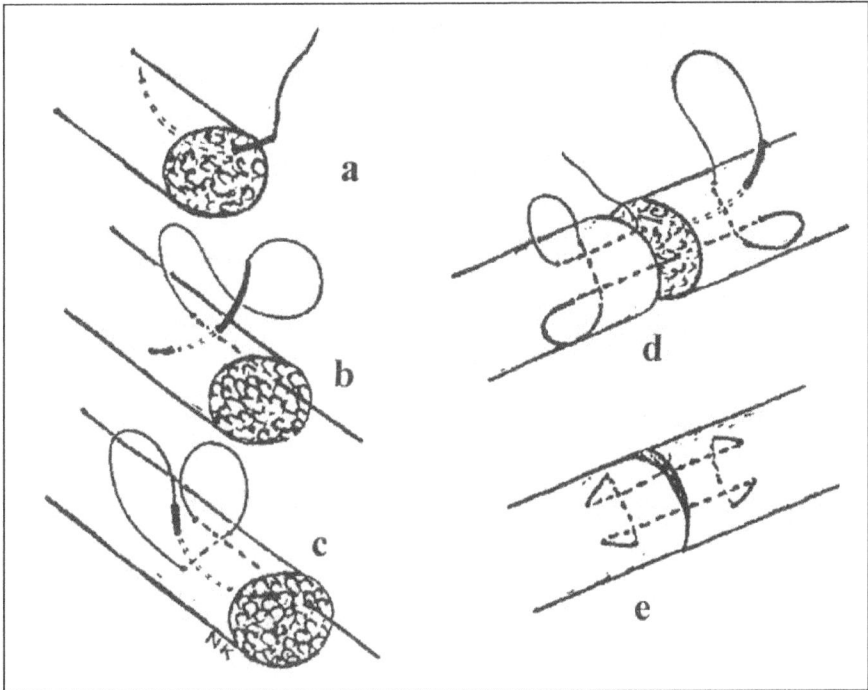

Figure 22.2: Locking Loop Technique.

Modified Kessler Technique

Same as locking loop technique except that in this technique the knot is secured on the out side of one of the tendon segments. Advantage- knot is outside the cut surface, hence no interference at the healing site.

Double Locking Loop Technique

Same as locking loop, except that instead of one loop, two loops are used so that there is increase in total number of sutures (4) crossing the site. Advantage-increase in strength.

Triple Locking Loop Technique

Three loops of suture materials are formed, so that 6 No. of sutures are crossed at the site. Advantage-gives more strength than single and double locking loop.

Three Loop Pulley Technique

Suture is passed in a near and far pattern comprising three loops, each of which is oriented approximately 120° from the other two loops. Advantage-provides greater strength and resistance to gap formation between the cut ends of the tendon.

Interrupted Mattress Suture Pattern

Interrupted horizontal mattress sutures are applied. Advantage-most suitable for flat tendons.

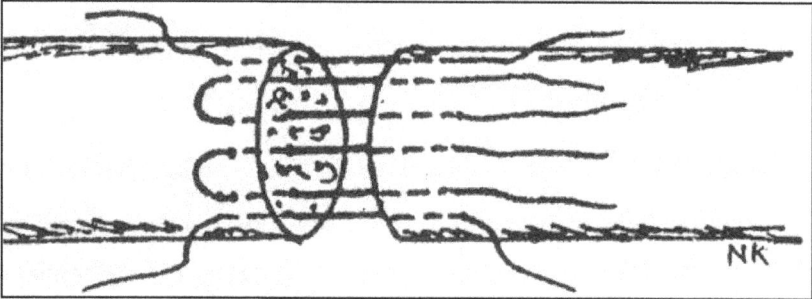

Figure 22.3: Interrupted Mattress Suture Pattern.

Overlapping Technique

Side to side anastomosis, fish mouth anastomosis. Advantage-provides stronger anastomosis. Disadvantage-requires greater tendon length, increases the diameter of final anastomosis.

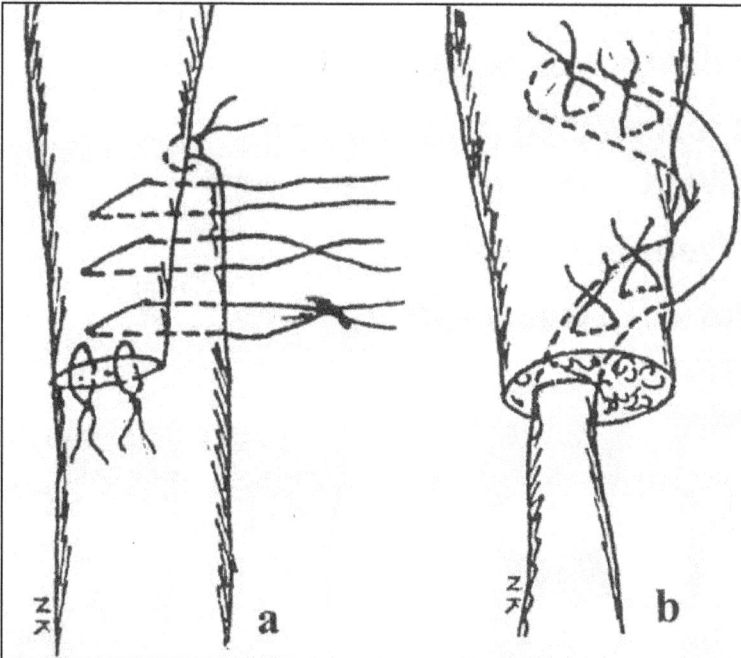

Figure 22.4: Overlapping Technique.

Tendon Lengthening Techniques

☆ Z-tenotomy

☆ Accordian technique

☆ Oblique section and gliding technique

☆ Lange technique

Tendon Shortening Techniques

☆ Doubling over method

☆ Z-tenotomy and segment excision

Contracted Tendons

Malformations of the extremities or parts of them are varied in their manifestations, ranging from absence of a single structure to partial or complete absence of the limbs. Congenital flexural deformities are seen within 1-2 weeks of birth. Contracted flexor tendon is a common abnormality of the musculoskeletal system in ruminants especially calves, and is caused by an autosomal recessive gene. The front limbs are primarily affected. In severe cases there may be some bony involvement, the condition is usually bilateral. An in utero positioning may also affect the degree of disability. At birth, the pastern and fetlocks of the forelegs and sometimes the carpal joints are flexed to varying degrees due to shortening of

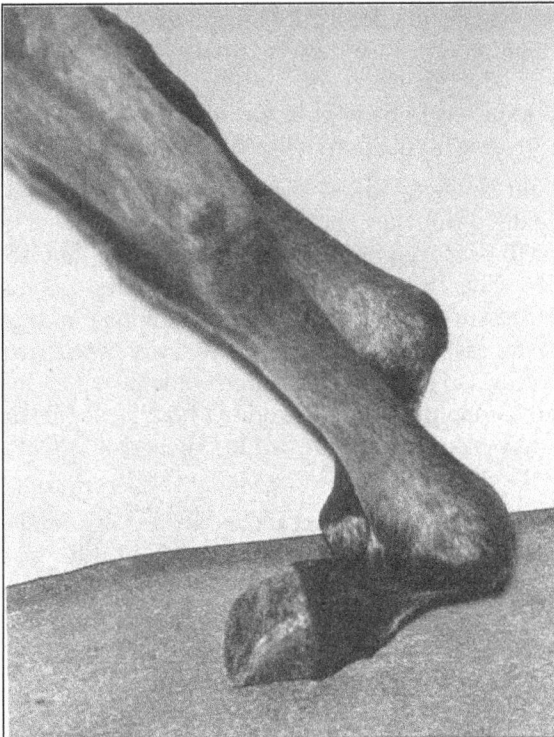

Figure 22.5: Contracted Tendons in a Calf.

the deep and superficial digital flexors and associated muscles. Slightly affected animals bear weight on the soles of the feet and walk on their toes. If not corrected, a septic arthritis of the fetlock joints is the usual sequel.

In newborn calves/foals, contraction or shortening of the flexor tendons results in knuckling of the fetlock joint frequently and of carpal joint rarely. The degree may vary from slight knuckling of the knee to complete flexion of the pastern and fetlock joints which rest on the ground. These symptoms are observed within the first one to two weeks after birth. Knuckling is usually observed in fore limbs and rarely hind limbs may be involved. Shortening of the digital flexors may be associated with other congenital abnormalities, such as cleft palate and arthrogryposis. Besides heritable factors, abnormal posture of the foetus in the uterus may be a predisposing factor. Trauma may be responsible for acquired nature of this condition in later life.

In mild contractions, a calf with slightly flexed fetlock joint stands and is able to walk on its toes without touching its heels on the ground. In advanced cases, the fetlock joint cannot be extended and the animal either stumbles or falls when it is made to walk. In more severe cases, the affected animal rests the dorsal aspect of the pastern or fetlock or both joints on the ground. Excoriation of the skin may lead to joint infection.

Treatment

In some calves, the flexion deformity improves spontaneously. In mild cases, treatment is not required because daily normal walking exercise is sufficient to stretch the tendons, which corrects the condition in due course of time. In other cases, the affected joint has to be kept in forced extension by a splint or a plaster cast to induce the inverse myotatic reflex with relaxation of the flexor muscles.

The limb should be well padded and the splint applied to the caudal aspect. The splint should extend from just above the foot to the elbow or hock. The support enables the animal to bear weight on toes and to use the limb so as to stretch the tendons gradually. The splint may be removed after 1-3 days to check for complications like pressure sores and oedema. Following massage, the splints may be reapplied. A plaster cast can also be used for two weeks so as to keep the tendons in a relaxed position and to allow the animal to walk normally. In severe cases or if above methods fail, a tenotomy of either one or both flexors is done and the limb immobilized. In a few cases, desmotomy of the suspensory ligament may become necessary.

For tenotomy, the animal is sedated and controlled in lateral recumbency with the affected limb lowermost. After local anaesthesia of the site, a skin incision is made on the medial aspect of the limb and parallel to the tendon. A mid metacarpal or metatarsal site is preferred where the tendon lacks the synovial sheath. The subcutaneous tissues are separated by blunt dissection, and the blood vessels are identified and retracted. Both tendons are identified and separated by blunt dissection. The affected tendon is transected while forcibly extending the fetlock joint. The skin wound is then sutured routinely. The gap between the two retracted ends of the tendon will fill with fibrous tissue. Z-tenotomy for lengthening tendon is an alternative technique for correction of the contracted tendons. A longitudinal incision is made in the center of the exposed tendon. At each end of the incision, a transverse incision is made but in opposite direction. The ends are then sutured. The skin incision is closed. The wound is protected by sterile bandage and a plaster cast then applied.

23

Teat Surgery

Mozammel Hoque

The udder and teat are vulnerable to external trauma or injury because of their anatomical location, increase in size of the udder and teat during lactation, faulty methods of milking, repeated trauma to the teat mucosa, injury by teeth of calf, unintentionally stepped teat, and paralysis resulting from the metabolic disturbances at parturition. Though teat surgery appears to be of minor in nature, it poses a great challenge to the dairy practitioner because of its glandular nature. Teat surgery is a demanding test of the skill of the surgeons. It demands proper surgical management and good aftercare that can save valuable animals from loosing one or more quarters or being culled.

Anatomy

Mammary glands are modified skin glands. In cows and buffaloes the mammary glands consists of four quarters. The glandular tissue of the udder is divided into two main halves-right and left, by a complete septum. The suspensory apparatus, and blood and nerve supplies of the two halves are independent of each other. Each half consists of a cranial and caudal quarter. The two quarters of each half have independent glandular tissue but common blood and nerve supply, and lymph drainage. The teats are membranous tubes consisting of skin, muscular layer (superficial longitudinal and deep circular fashion), fibrous layer and mucosa. The closing mechanism of the teat consists of circular muscles forming the sphincter, the rosette of Furstenberg and circular elastic fibres around the streak canal. In sheep, the udder consists of two halves with one teat each, and each half resembles one quarter of bovine udder.

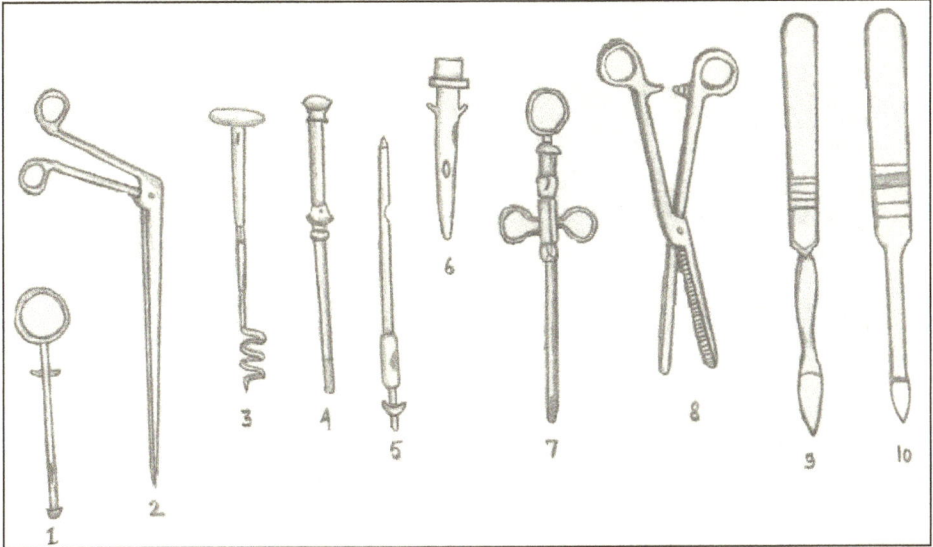

Figure 23.1: Commonly Used Teat Instruments.
1. Hug's teat tumour extractor, 2. Alligator forceps, 3. Hudson's teat spiral, 4. Teat dilator, 5. Teat siphon, 6. Larson's teat tube, 7. Three-ring teat slitter 8. Small artery forceps, 9. Lichy teat knife-blunt point,10. Lichy teat knife-sharp point.

Restraint and Anaesthesia

Animal may be restrained within a crate with one leg lifted.

Local anaesthesia at the teat base with or without sedation and with the animal in lateral recumbency.

Xylazine alone is effective for minor procedure, but contraindicated in advanced gestation and possible recumbency.

Diagnosis

☆ History and clinical examination

☆ Probing with sterilized teat siphon

☆ Radiography- positive contrast and double contrast radiography are used to detect structural teat abnormalities.

☆ Ultrasonography- used to detect the level and extent of obstruction, depth of laceration and echo-intensity of udder tissue.

☆ Theloscopy- teat endoscopy, is a useful technique for diagnosis and therapy of covered teat injuries.

Preparation for Surgery

Withholding feed and water for 12-24 hrs when surgery is done in recumbent position. Cleaning and washing of udder and teat with antiseptic solution.

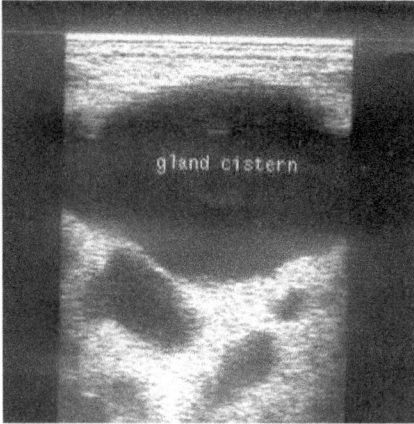

Figure 23.2: Sonogram of Gland Cistern.

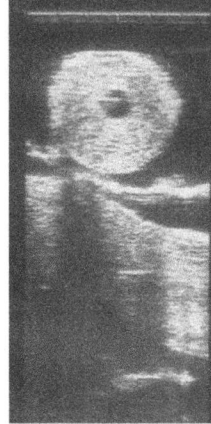

Figure 23.3: Sonogram of Obstructed Teat.

Surgical Diseases

Some common forms of surgical affections are laceration, fistula, obstruction, stenosis and thelitis.

Supernumerary Teats

Congenital and inherited condition. Small teats are commonly caudal, but sometimes are attached to the normal teat. Remove when 1-9 months old, and never within 1 month of parturition as it may lead to oedema, wound dehiscence, infection and mastitis. Crush at the base with small Burdizzo and resect with knife along the inner edge of blades. Line of section should be cranial to caudal, not transverse so that subsequent scar merges into natural folds of udder skin. Suture only if wound edges separate. Alternative technique is to remove surgically under local analgesia by making two elliptical incisions at the junction of the teat and skin of the udder. The wound is closed with interrupted sutures using a non absorbable suture material.

Teat Lacerations

Incidence of teat laceration is relatively higher in goats due to their pendulous udder and long teats. Superficial wounds are treated as standard with other tissues. Large wound involving skin and muscularis may require suturing. Deep wound involving mucosa is best sutured with the animal in lateral recumbency after deep sedation. A ring block is produced and a tourniquet is applied at the base of the teat to check haemorrhage and to prevent milk flow into the cistern. After preparation of the affected teat, a sterilized teat siphon is inserted and debridement is done to remove the dead tissue. The mucosa is closed with simple continuous/ interrupted suture with absorbable suture material. The submucosa and muscularis are then closed together using simple continuous suture and finally the skin is closed. Post-operatively antibiotics are infused into the affected teat for 4-5 days.

Milk is removed after insertion of a sterile teat siphon for a few days for smooth haling.

Teat Fistula

Teat fistula is an abnormal opening between the teat cistern and the teat surface through which milk flows out in lactating animals. If the fistula is very small, mild chemical cauterization or electric cautery may be helpful. Large fistula needs reconstructive surgery. Surgery should be delayed if the teat is highly inflamed. For repair, two elliptical incisions are given on the skin edges for debridement and undermining. The wound is then closed as mentioned earlier for deep lacerations.

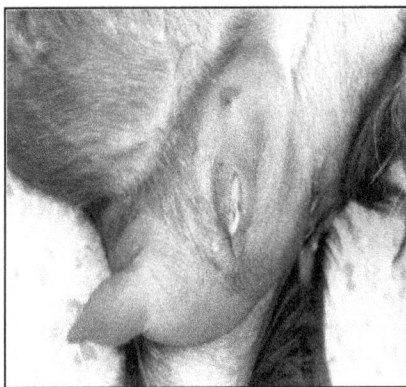

Figure 23.4: Teat Fistula Before Surgery.

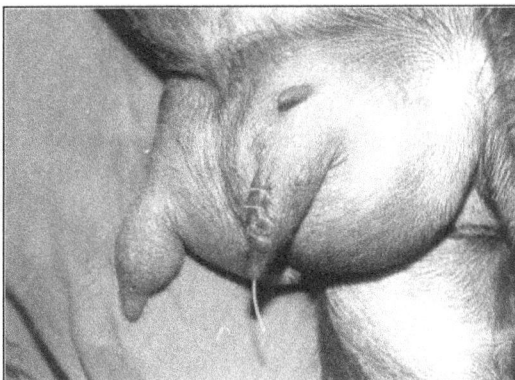

Figure 23.5: Teat Fistula After Surgery.

Teat Spider (Membranous Obstruction)

May be congenital or acquired. The obstructing membrane may be thick or thin and located high at the base of the teat or lower down in the cistern. Palpation shows fluctuating milk above the obstructions but milking is not possible. The teat is prepared for surgery under local analgesia. A Hudson's teat spiral is introduced up to the membrane for deep penetration with 3-4 revolutions, and the instrument is then withdrawn. Alternatively, the membrane can be slit in 3-4 directions using a small teat bistoury. Flow of the milk generally keeps the teat cistern patent. It is recommended during milking not to milk the affected quarter completely to avoid a stricture.

Contracted Sphincter (Hard Milker)

It may be congenital or acquired. There is a small stream of milk leading to prolonged milking time and trauma to the teat.

Under local analgesia, the enlarging procedure may be accomplished by inserting a Litchy teat knife, ringed teat slitter or Stoll teat bistoury. The opening in the sphincter is maintained at the desired size by inserting a Larson teat tube and leaving it in place for 5-7 days. Milking is accomplished by removing the cap of the tube.

Free Milker or Leaker (Enlarged Teat Orifice)

Milk leaks from the teat at times other than milking due to a relaxed or traumatized sphincter. Injection of minute amount of sterile mineral oil or Lugol's solution using a 22-26 G hypodermic needle around the orifice may help to reduce its size to the desired level. This may have to be done more than once to obtain the optimal size for milk flow.

Imperforate Teat (Occlusion of Teat Orifice)

May be congenital or acquired. For treatment, an 18 G hypodermic needle is forced into the teat cistern under local analgesia. Once the milk starts coming out, the teat orifice is treated as mentioned for contracted orifice.

Lactolith (Milk Stone)

Lactoliths in the teat cistern form due to mineral deposits and may interfere in milking. Small lactoliths can be removed by milking them out through the teat orifice. A mosquito forceps can be used to crush a large lactolith and then small pieces can be removed by milking. If the lactoliths are hard and large, the sphincter may be slit and removed.

Papilloma (Warts)

They are finger like projections originate from the skin surface of the teat. A tight ligature at the base of the wart is applied to drop off it or surgically removed.

Polyps

Generally pea sized growth attached to the wall of the teat cistern, which interferes with milk flow. A teat tumour extractor, a curette or a teat polyp extractor may be used to remove the growth.

Thelitis

Acute or per acute inflammatory condition of one or more teats, which is distinct from infectious mastitis where culture of milk samples shows no pathological bacteria. Intralesional methylprednisolone and hyaluronidase along with systemic antibiotic and antihistamine drugs provide superior results.

Amputation of Mammary Gland

Indicated in gangrenous mastitis. General anaesthesia or epidural block is used. For unilateral gland amputation, the incision is placed at the superiolateral aspect of the gland about 2-3 cm away from the intermammary groove. For bilateral amputation, incision should start at the midline caudally near the base of the udder to extend cranially along the base. The skin is resected from both edges. One of the glands is dissected away from the line of cutaneous incision to expose the external pudic artery and vein located near the external inguinal ring. Similarly, reflection of the cranial part of the gland will expose the perineal artery and large subcutaneous vein. All the vessels should be doubly ligated with a strong absorbable suture material. If both glands need removal, the procedure is repeated on the other gland. The skin flaps are closed.

Recent Trends in Teat Surgery

Ultrasonography facilitates accurate diagnosis of pathological conditions which are sometime impossible to detect by clinical examination. Linear or sector transducers of 5-10 MHz have been used for the purpose. This non invasive technique enables clinician to detect the level and extent of abnormalities within the canals, sinus and glandular tissue of the gland. The udder and teat are amenable to sonographic imaging because of its superficial location and has the potential to diagnose different conditions of the organ.

Endoscopy is a new, modern method used in the diagnosis and therapy of the teat disorders. Two methods of teat endoscopy can be used: endoscopy through the teat canal or endoscopy from the side access (through the wall of the teat). Apart from visualization of inaccessible organs, endoscopy enables surgical operations within the teat canal. This method necessitates the use of the theloresectoscope (length 150 mm, diameter 2.7 mm), cold light source, fiber optic light cable, endoflator and cold light source, fiber optic light cable, endoflator and trocar. Theloscopy using an endoscope has been proven quicker, less invasive, atraumatic, and free of major post-operative complications such as haemorrhages, inefficient wound healing and mastitis. Most of the currently applied techniques for mammary gland endoscopy have curative purposes and focus on treatment of teat injuries and stenosis in high yielding dairy cows.

Low level laser therapy effects healing of teat and udder wounds by minimizing inflammation, improvement of skin regeneration and enhancement of collagen synthesis.

Open teat surgery is the surgical procedure of cutting through the teat wall to enable the surgeon to correct problems in the teat or udder cistern. By this approach the surgeon can visualize the problem and exercise sound surgical judgement in correcting it. This is superior to blind ripping and cutting through the streak canal. Correct suturing of the incision in layers is most important. Provision of drainage is also recommended.

Silicone implant and NIT natural teat inserts have been used to keep the teat canal patent after surgery.

Index

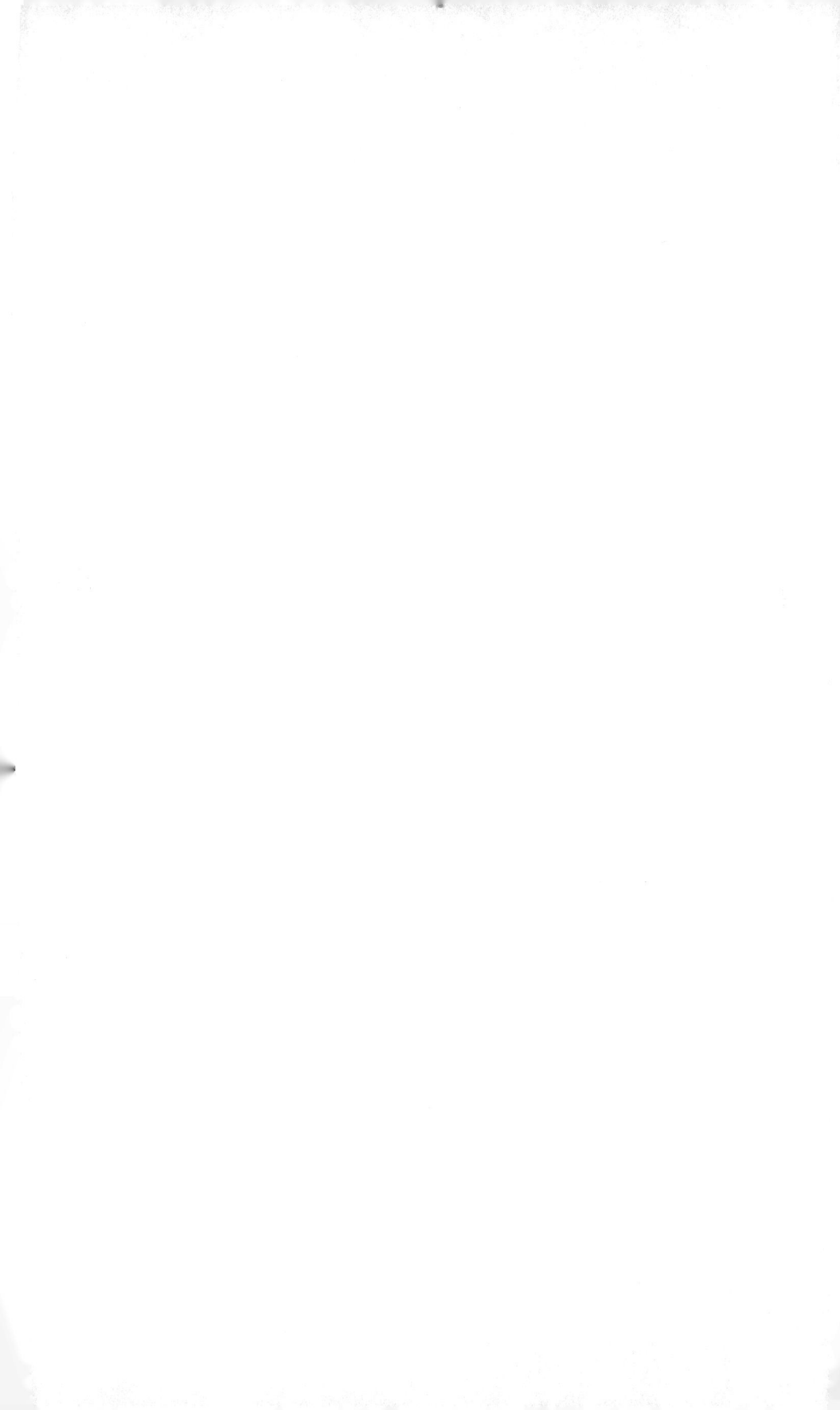

www.ingramcontent.com/pod-product-compliance
Lightning Source LLC
Chambersburg PA
CBHW021434180326
41458CB00001B/270